Yoga Bodies

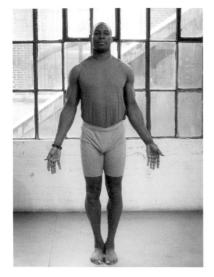
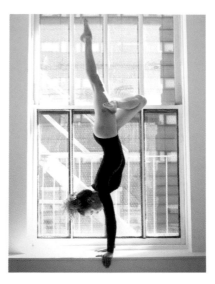
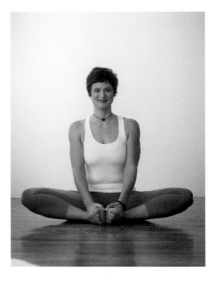
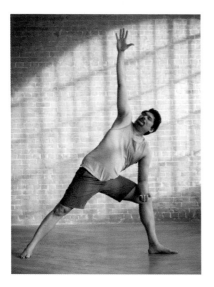
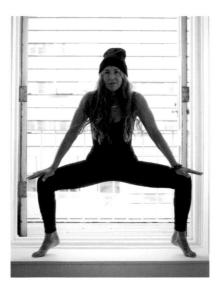
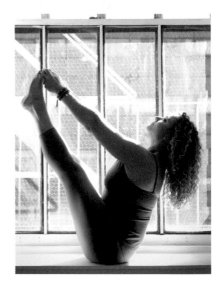
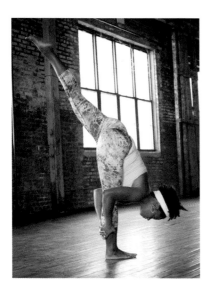
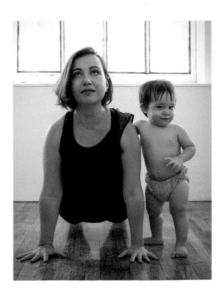
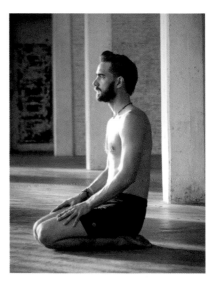

Yoga Bodies

Real People, Real Stories
& the Power of Transformation

LAUREN LIPTON
PHOTOGRAPHS BY JAIMIE BAIRD

CHRONICLE BOOKS
SAN FRANCISCO

Library of Congress Cataloging-in-Publication Data

Names: Lipton, Lauren, 1966-
Title: Yoga bodies : real people, real stories, and the power of transformation / Lauren Lipton ;
    photographs by Jaimie Baird.
Description: San Francisco : Chronicle Books, [2017]
Identifiers: LCCN 2016025949 | ISBN 9781452156033 (hardback)
Subjects: LCSH: Hatha yoga—Popular works. | Self-care, Health—Popular
    works. | BISAC: SELF-HELP / Personal Growth / Happiness. | HEALTH & FITNESS / Yoga.
Classification: LCC RA781.7 .L57 2017 | DDC 613.7/046—dc23 LC record available at
https://lccn.loc.gov/2016025949

Manufactured in China

Design by Anne Kenady

The information, practices, and poses in this book are not offered as medical advice or
suggested as treatment for any condition that might require medical attention. To avoid
injury, practice yoga with a skilled instructor and consult a health professional to determine
your body's needs and limitations. The author, photographer, and publisher hereby disclaim
any liability from injuries resulting from following any recommendation in this book.

10 9 8 7 6 5 4 3 2 1

Chronicle Books LLC
680 Second Street
San Francisco, California 94107
www.chroniclebooks.com

TO JAMES

Namaste

INTRODUCTION

This book is for every yogi.

It is for lifelong yogis, for yogis newer to the practice, and for yogis who have never stepped foot on a mat. That is, who haven't *yet*.

If you've tried yoga, you may have experienced what I call the yoga buzz. Leaving the studio after class, maybe you found yourself unexpectedly happy, thinking, "Everything is exactly as it should be." In this enchanted state, the world, even with its suffering, heartache, and aggravation, feels miraculous. People seem divine and beautiful, and you remember that despite our disagreements, we're all traveling through life with one another for company. The feeling doesn't last forever; inevitably, honking horns and arguments and "your call is very important to us" sneak back in to mess with your yoga buzz. But you can get it back whenever you want, just by returning to your mat.

The wish that everybody might have access to this deeply peaceful state of mind led me to create this book.

Yoga Bodies celebrates the many ways yoga can bring joy and meaning to our lives and demonstrates that anyone can do it. You don't have to be athletic and flexible, or any particular age, shape, or size (or, as you'll discover in these pages, even human). You don't need to embrace Eastern spirituality or chant in Sanskrit. You need not wear yoga pants, eat kale, or spend years perfecting your poses—or, in Sanskrit, *asanas*. There's no rule that you have to say "*asana*."

You definitely don't have to have a "yoga body," at least not in the ungenerous way the media often defines it: sexy, skinny, and able to contort into impossible positions. The superstar yogis you see in magazines and on the Internet, the women and men who backbend on paddleboards and handstand on cliffs, are extraordinary talents. Some of them are in this book. And they would be the first to tell you that they don't own the term "yoga body." They believe,

6

as does anyone who has absorbed the lessons of yoga, that *every* body is a yoga body. Already. We're born that way.

By the same notion, there is no single definition of yoga. As you'll see in this book, yoga invites each of us to define it as we wish.

To me, yoga is the practice of observing myself exactly as I am right now, with no specific expectation of what will happen in the future—whether that's one second, a week, or twenty years from now. The poses figure in because they keep my mind busy as I work to, say, hold Half Moon Pose. There's so much to focus on—Gaze toward the ceiling! Keep breathing! Stay upright!—that my anxious mind, which is usually very busy regaling me with a kaleidoscope of catastrophes that might befall me, falls silent. That tiny, temporary respite feels like a vacation. (By the way, although I have been practicing yoga for a while, I am still not great at having no expectations and no anxiety. But I'm getting better.)

So that's how I see yoga, but my definition is by no means the official or only one. In this book you'll find a different interpretation of yoga with each turn of the page, as more than eighty people express, in words and poses, what yoga means to them.

The yogis in this book are on their own journeys. A few are beginners; some teach yoga for a living. If you know your yoga, you may spot some imperfect poses. That's also part of the message of *Yoga Bodies*. Each of these images, by photographer Jaimie Baird, captures one yogi in one pose at one moment in time that is now long past. "Perfection," if it even exists, is elusive.

But each of these yogis is divine and beautiful. So are you. So is everyone. We're in this together. We are all yoga bodies.

—Lauren Lipton

Twee

BOUND TRIANGLE POSE

...

My name is actually spelled "Thuy." I changed it to a phonetic spelling after college so it would be easier for people to understand.

My family came to America from Vietnam at the end of the Vietnam War. I was five. My father was an Irish-American who worked in Vietnam for an American company. My mother, who is Vietnamese, worked in my father's office. From what my parents told us, as my mom was collecting the papers for us to leave Vietnam, she had to run in between buildings while explosions were happening in the background.

I don't remember much of Vietnam from my childhood. Our parents had servants and nannies there, but here they worked their butts off. My mom had to learn English. They were both pretty much in survival mode. My sister once told me we were on food stamps for a while back then. I was like, "We were?"

We four siblings took care of each other, which was fun. But things were definitely not fine. In fourth grade, three boys would tease me and call me "chink." I would have liked to be blond with blue eyes, the all-American girl.

It wasn't until I was in my thirties and went back to Vietnam with my mom that I finally started to let go of these ideas of who I wasn't. I was on the way to a cemetery to visit my great-uncle's grave, walking though a beautiful vast green rice field. Suddenly, I did this 360-degree *Sound of Music* thing where I was like, "I am Asian! I have slanted eyes, and I love it! This is who I am!"

Now I see differences between people, differences in our skin colors and our beliefs, but I think, "Who cares? We're all the same."

One of my yoga teachers explained it this way: Imagine a huge wax ball. That's consciousness. Pull a piece of it and stretch it out. Along the stretchiness of it, there are animals, plants, humans, all part of that invisible ball of consciousness.

When he said this, I was like, "Oh—it's all just God with different faces."

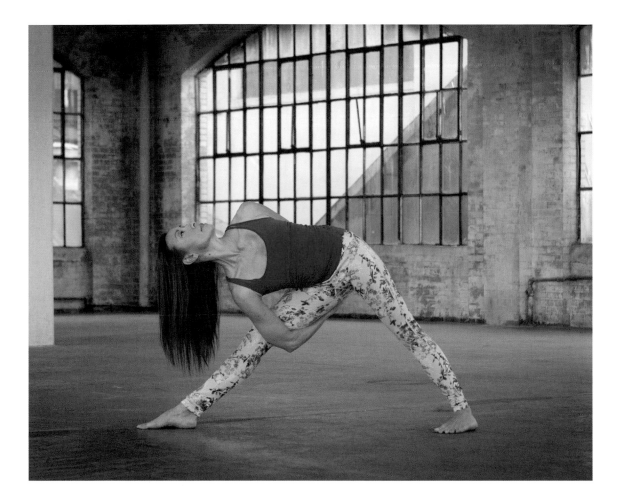

Margarita

SPHINX POSE

...

During labor with Pedro, I was able to use my yoga training to drop into my body and let it guide what I was doing. I had my eyes closed a lot of the time and was so focused on this internal experience. There was something incredible about it.

I found it strange and unexpected that I wanted to be upright. I was in active labor for about seven hours and was moving around pretty much the whole time. I walked the halls, or I stood and leaned forward against my partner. I wasn't necessarily trying to ease the pain, because there wasn't any getting away from that. I was just using movement to flow through it.

Some people call contractions "rushes" or "quickenings," which is a good way to reframe them in your mind. Contractions are a tightening. But labor is a loosening. You're trying to open and allow your body to birth. You have to relax, which is an ability we don't usually work on in our lives.

But it's important to practice. If I'm on the subway platform, waiting for the train, I'll often use those two minutes to consciously relax and slow down. This is also yoga, and it was a useful skill during labor. When I wasn't having contractions, I could bring my awareness to, "Right now I'm not in pain; I can relax. And at the end of all of this, I will have a beautiful baby."

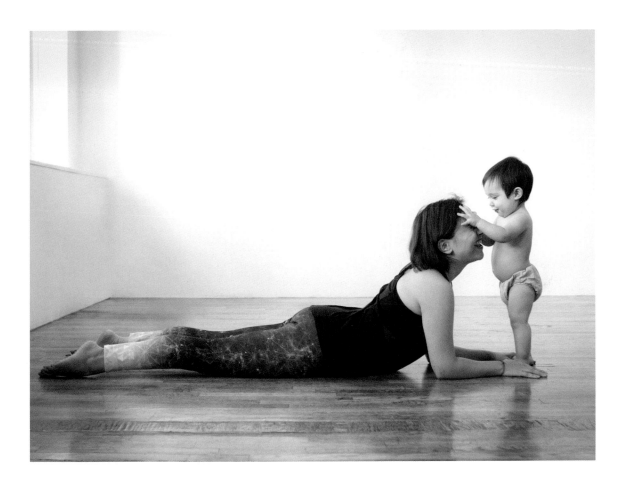

Alan

ACCOMPLISHED POSE

. . .

Since I began practicing asana and meditation at age sixteen, I must admit, I have missed only eight days. For two of those days I was very young and wanted to see how it felt not to practice. For another couple of those days I was laid up with hip surgery, and for a couple more my son was in the hospital. But besides those eight days, I have practiced yoga every day. As a result, I can go into *samadhi* at any time, in any place. If I couldn't, what would be the point of doing fifty-five years of yoga?

Samadhi is difficult to describe, but it is the state of having a still mind, of turning your senses inward. When you reach *samadhi*, you are in the now, where there's no form of duality—no separation between you and everything in the universe. There is no time, no form, no good or bad, light or dark, right or wrong. When I teach people to meditate, I teach them how to move their consciousness toward *samadhi*. So I like to say I teach people to feel nothing.

I can find *samadhi* on the bus, in the middle of the city, wherever. I was interviewed for a documentary a few years ago, and the interviewer asked me, "You can just go outside on the street and feel *samadhi*?" I said, "Let's go." We went down to Fifty-eighth Street and sat on a curb outside the Bloomberg building. People were walking by. For about two minutes I was unaware of New York City around me. I could have sat there for much longer, but I didn't want the crew to feel like they had to keep filming me.

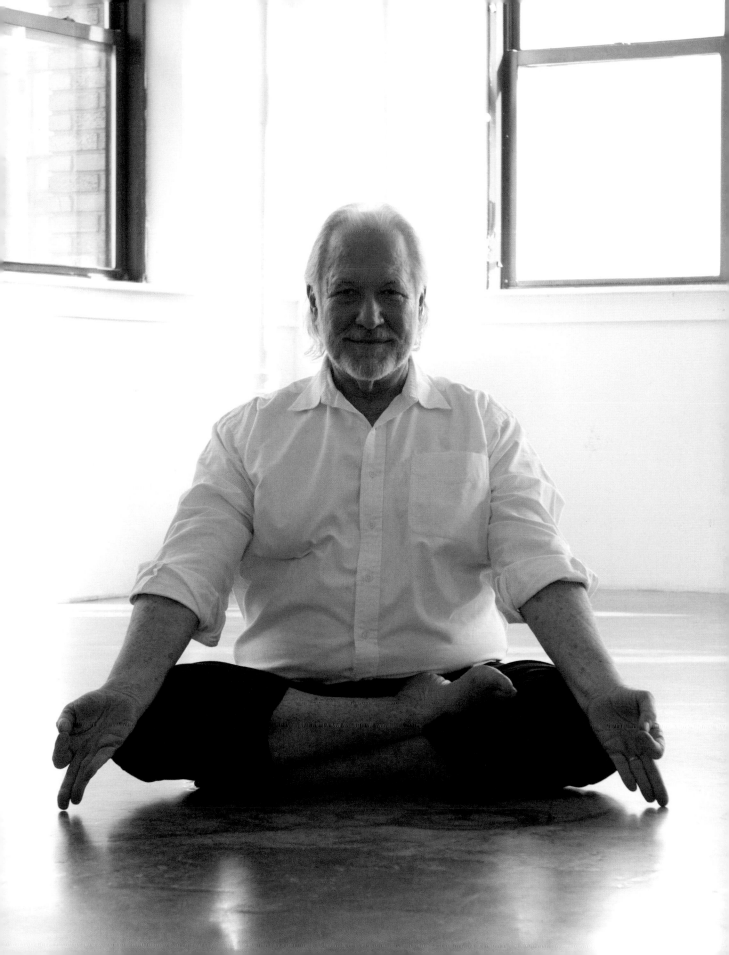

Kim

FROG POSE

...

When I first started practicing yoga, I used to be uncomfortable with the *Om*. Our teacher would have us chant it before and after class, and I would try to stop before everyone else did because I didn't want my voice to be the last one heard. I also wasn't sure what *Om* meant. Not that I'm such an observant Jew, but in the beginning I remember being led through *Om* and other, longer Sanskrit chants and wondering, "What am I saying? Does it contradict my Judaism?"

Now I understand that *Om* is really just a sound—a universal sound—and a vibration in your chest cavity. I like the way that vibration feels. It is an internal massage and it stretches my lungs. I find it very comforting, especially after the practice. I went from "I don't want to do this" to really looking forward to it, to wanting my voice to be heard.

I love chanting now. It turns out that it's very nice things you are saying. The singing and music is my favorite part of going to synagogue, and the Sanskrit chants are all the same stuff expressed in another way. They're about nature and intention and balance. *Om Shanti Shanti,* like *shalom*, is a call for peace. Another chant I love, *Om Namah Shivaya,* was more troubling for me at first because it is a prayer to the Hindu god Shiva, but I substitute a prayer to my inner self and to healing.

There's nothing in those chants that contradicts my Judaism. Instead, they add to it.

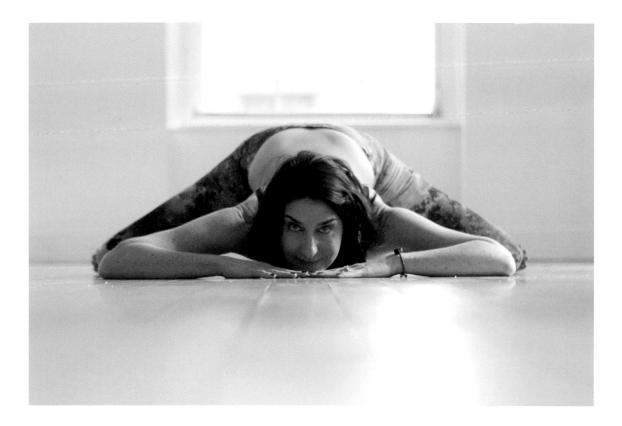

Jessamyn

CAMEL POSE VARIATION

...

After I had been involved in yoga for a while as a body-positive advocate, so many people told me, "You should go to teacher training," but I was like, "I'm not going to be a yoga teacher." There were too many yoga teachers already. Why did I need to be another one?

My father helped change how I saw all of this. He does not care about the weird world of Internet publicity and did not acknowledge my Internet presence—he still doesn't. But last year, I found myself in this big media bubble. I was on *Good Morning America* and in *New York* magazine. After I began to get mainstream attention, my dad said, "It seems like you need to do this, Jessamyn," and offered to pay for my teacher training.

It was the most incredible, life-changing experience I've ever had. I'm kind of the anti-yogi and maybe went into the training somewhat jaded. By the second week, I was, like, crying. I was doing a partner exercise with a girl a lot smaller than me. I kept apologizing for putting my body weight on her: "Oh, I'm sorry. Oh, I'm sorry. I'm sorry."

She finally said, "You know you don't have to apologize, right?"

I said, "I guess I'm apologizing for my own existence."

Then I thought, "Oh, my god, I really think that."

I cried all the way home. It was the most cleansing experience. I have issues with being fat. I have issues with my blackness. I apologize because I cannot accept my own existence. So many people feel the same way. I have told this story so many times, and someone always says, "I feel that."

That is the reason to teach yoga—to help others acknowledge these things and move past them.

The more people who are trained to be yoga teachers, the more people there are to spread around its messages. The training opened my heart, and it opened my eyes.

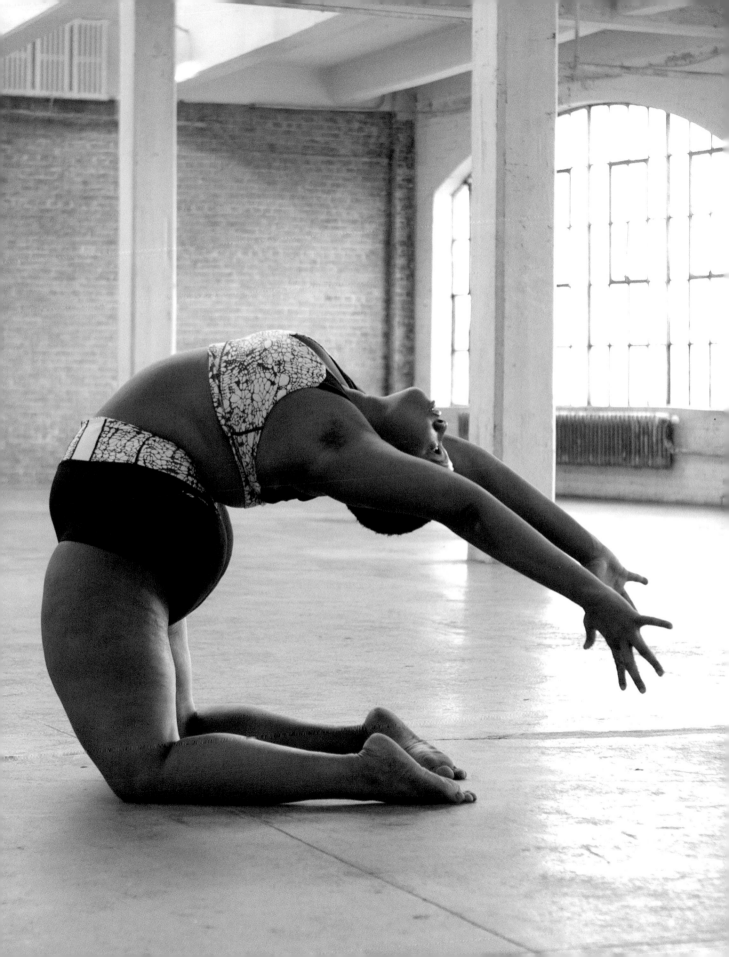

Betsy

MONKEY POSE

* * *

I fell off a cliff. I was twenty-six and traveling through northern Minnesota with a then-girlfriend to see the aurora borealis. We had booked a cabin for the weekend, and about halfway there we stopped at a scenic overlook called Gooseberry Falls. It's this beautiful vista where you can see for a huge expanse and look down onto a canyon where a river cuts through to form a series of waterfalls.

My girlfriend was a photographer and wanted to take some photos, so we decided to walk down the trail for a bit. We had probably walked for ten minutes when the sky opened up and it started to pour down rain. We ran at full speed to get back to the car. I was wearing a miniskirt and brand-new cowboy boots, and I slipped on a slimy rock and slid right off the edge of the trail.

The fall was thirty feet, straight down. There wasn't even a slope.

People always ask me, "Did you have visions of your whole life flashing before your eyes?" I didn't. I had been reading the novel *The Unbearable Lightness of Being.* What went through my head as I was falling was, "Become unbearably light." I had an image of how a feather falls, wafting from side to side. I thought, "Be unbearably light, and land like a feather."

I landed on a rock slab. If it had not been there, I would have fallen another forty feet into the river and all of the waterfalls. All that happened was I got a sprained ankle and tore a ligament and cartilage in my knee.

You might think, "That must have sucked." But that fall woke me up in a big way. The moment I landed, I felt more like, "I'm so lucky to be alive." I didn't start doing yoga until much later, but I understood right then that I needed to figure out how to be more present and really appreciate my life. That's the moment the yogi in me was born.

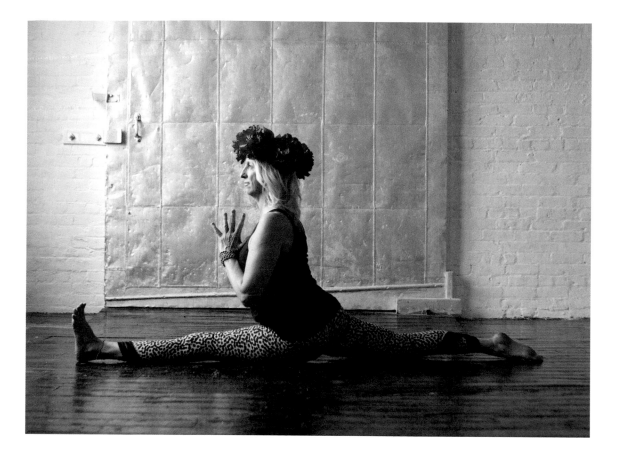

Babette

COW FACE POSE VARIATION

...

Aging is totally uncelebrated in our society. I wish there was some way to change the attitude of Western culture toward aging and the aged. Because it's so stupid to try to fight it. We all get there—we all age. You can't do anything except to stay as healthy and mindful as possible, and to try to get as much as you can out of life. Am I at peace with aging? Nobody is at peace with aging, if they're honest about it.

The majority of people at a lot of yoga studios are young. I mean *young.* I took a three-day workshop recently, and half the people in there were decades younger than I am. At my usual studio, there's a wonderful age range. Still, at seventy-eight, I'm the oldest person in the room, for sure.

It doesn't bother me at all. I'm just used to it. If everybody in the entire room is twenty-two, they might look at me sort of weirdly when I walk in, but I am more self-conscious about how I look as an older person when I'm in front of my own mirror at home and I see that my skin isn't the way it was twenty or thirty years ago.

But when I'm doing yoga, I don't even think about that.

Everyone's whole body is changing all the time. It isn't the same between the left and the right sides, between morning and evening, between today and Thursday. What happens to me—and this might be age and it might not—is that I find that just because I've nailed a pose doesn't mean I can do it every time. Some days I can do pose X but not pose Y, and some days I can do Y but not X. Some days I can do both, and some days I can do neither.

You learn in yoga to be able to say, "Yeah, today my balance is terrible. Yesterday my balance was wonderful." You can accept these things, instead of saying, "I did this yesterday; why can't I do it today?" You can't do it today because your body is different today.

And it doesn't matter. I don't mean this as a platitude, and I'm far from a Pollyanna. But whatever you are is what you have. That's what is. You might as well allow it to be OK.

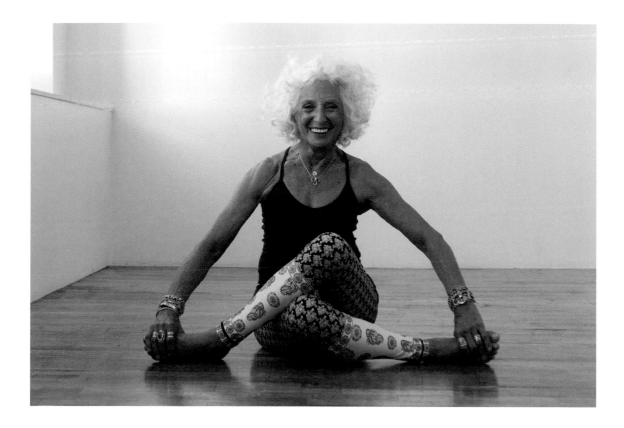

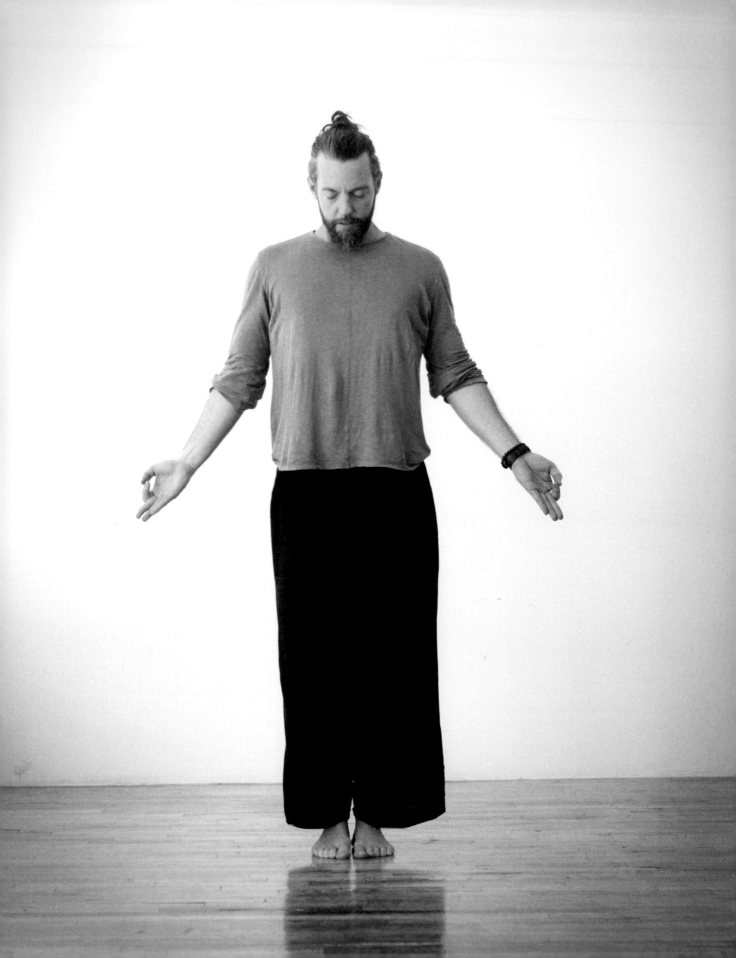

Kevin

MOUNTAIN POSE VARIATION

. . .

In the late 1990s, during the whole dot-com era, I worked for an Internet start-up. I was making really good money, and then the company went public, and I went on that whole ride. The stock price shot up, I had all these shares, and with this perceived wealth, I felt like, "I've really gotten somewhere. I'm really arriving." A few months later the stock tanked and it all totally dissolved. I would rather not say specifically how much I lost, but let's just say it went from a lot to me cashing out at the end of it all with a few thousand dollars.

That, and other painful losses around the same time, catalyzed me. My overriding thinking was, "I have to make a change." I decided to pursue my love for yoga and become a teacher. Not long after, I decided to go live in Thailand and devote myself to deeper studies. I felt that I needed to be far away and fully immersed in it so I could get clear. I wanted to be breathing and conscious and awake.

I was brought up in a system where the expectations are that you go to college, get a job, buy a house, and start a family. It turned out that I wanted something totally different.

I'm back in the North American cultural paradigm now and still very much have pursuits in which I want to be successful, but I live a more holistic, fully engaged life. Now I work with corporate executives to awaken them to the idea that they don't have to go all the way to a remote mountaintop to find and live a life of clarity, truth, and authenticity.

Marsha

TREE POSE

...

I was diagnosed with bone cancer when I was five years old. I had chemotherapy and radiation. Then, when I was thirteen, it happened again. The cancer came back in the exact same location, and that's when I had the amputation.

I also had more, pretty aggressive chemo. The job of chemotherapy is to kill things, and it killed my kidneys. Twenty years after the chemo, when I was thirty-three, my kidneys just stopped working, and I had to start going in for dialysis.

In dialysis, a machine does what your kidneys normally do: It cleans your blood, removing waste and chemicals. You're hooked up through tubing connected to two needles in your arm. The blood runs through one tube and is processed through a filter, and the clean blood is returned to your body through the other tube. The process takes up a lot of your life. Each session lasts four hours in the hospital, and for the rest of the day I would be zonked. But if your kidneys fail and you want to be alive, you have to do dialysis. If you don't, you can be dead really quickly.

So I did this every Monday, Wednesday, and Friday for eleven years, until I finally got a kidney transplant.

The thing with dialysis is that everything is right there on the surface for you to watch. Your life depends on a machine, and you can see the machine in front of you, literally removing your blood and washing it. It's pretty unbelievable and amazing, like a fast river moving.

I had done some yoga on and off, but it was in dialysis that I had this miraculous calling to help people understand that they're never separate from their essence, and that their essence is really this divine energy. You can be as close to death as I was and have this *prana,* this life force, flowing through you.

I don't think I would have as much empathy if all of these things hadn't happened to me. Everybody has their story. Everybody has their losses. We've all had something brutally cut off from us in some way. We all have to go through that process of recovery.

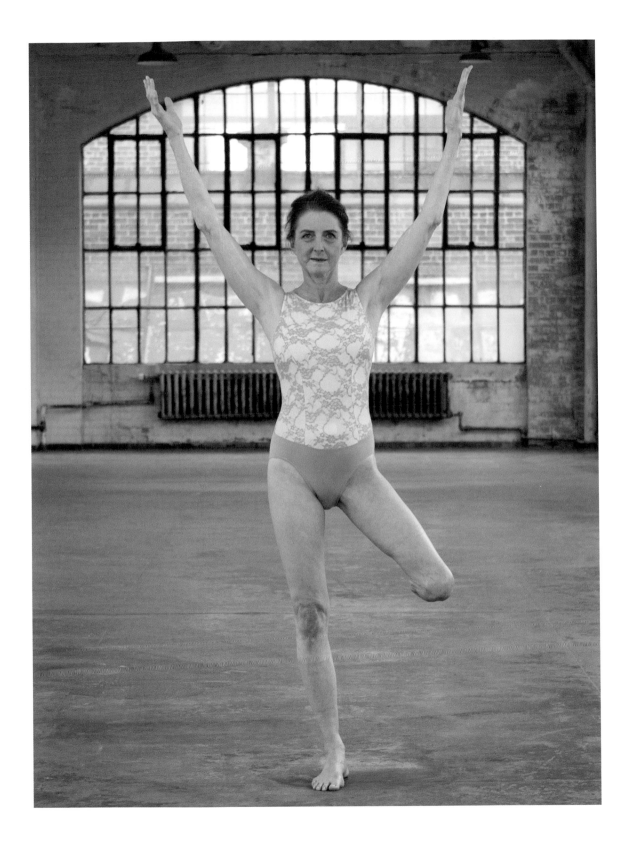

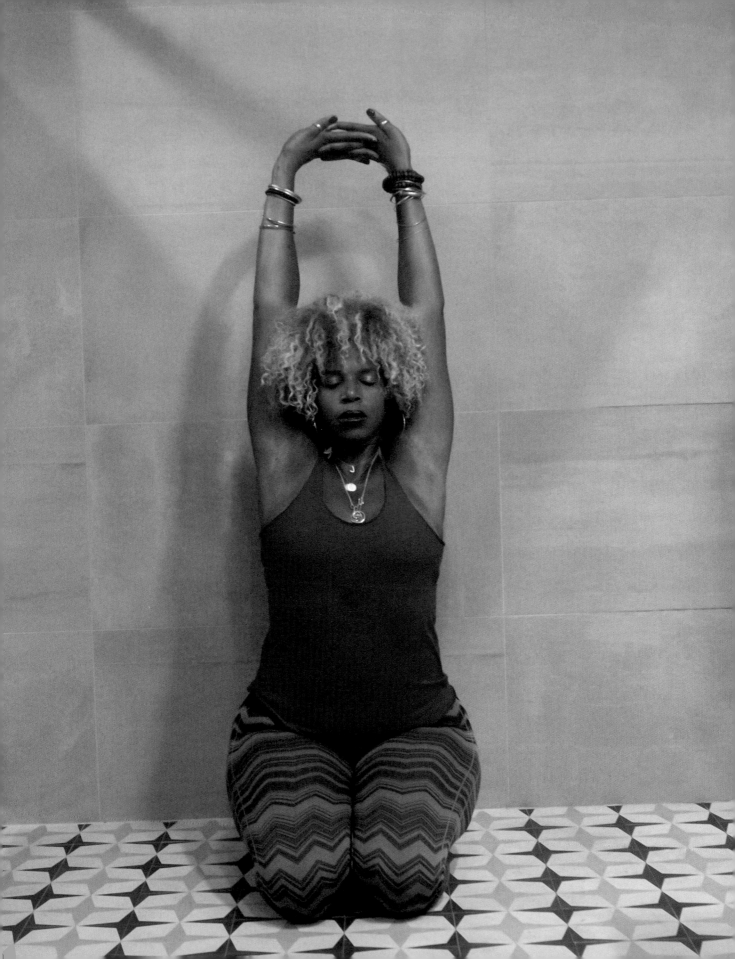

Jyll

DIAMOND POSE VARIATION

...

One reason I do yoga is so I don't punch somebody in the throat. When I was younger, I would get so angry I would have nosebleeds. Inconsiderate people, liars, people who are self-absorbed—they're the worst. I do yoga so when I'm confronted with somebody like that I can stop, count to ten, and say, "How may I help you?" I'm still getting there, but it's definitely easier. I can let things roll now.

A few months ago I was at a party with my husband. I was in heels and had my hair wrapped up. We got into an elevator with some white people, and this guy said to me, "What's up, Aunt Jemima?"

He was about twenty-five and drunk, and after he said it, he realized what he'd done. He said, "That was inappropriate, right? OK. What's up, sista?"

I could feel the walls of that elevator caving in on me. It was one of the most humiliating experiences I have ever been through. I kept waiting for my husband to step up to the plate and handle it, but he did not. I am over six feet tall in my heels and could have easily taken the guy out, but I didn't; this was a work event for my husband. As soon as the elevator doors opened, I ran out and started crying. I tried to let things roll, but even with all the yoga I've done, I couldn't help my state of mind right then.

That little racial incident really hurt. I have tried to let it go, but it still lingers in the back of my mind. You know what it is? That's just not how I live my life. My community is diverse and politically correct. My husband is Jewish; we've got three biracial kids. My brother is married to his white partner. I don't have things like that happen to me, so when it did, I was shook. Even when I talk about it now, it still shakes me.

Sometimes I wonder what that scene in the elevator would have been like if I didn't have yoga in my life. I'm sure it would have been different. Who knows? It could have been a lot worse.

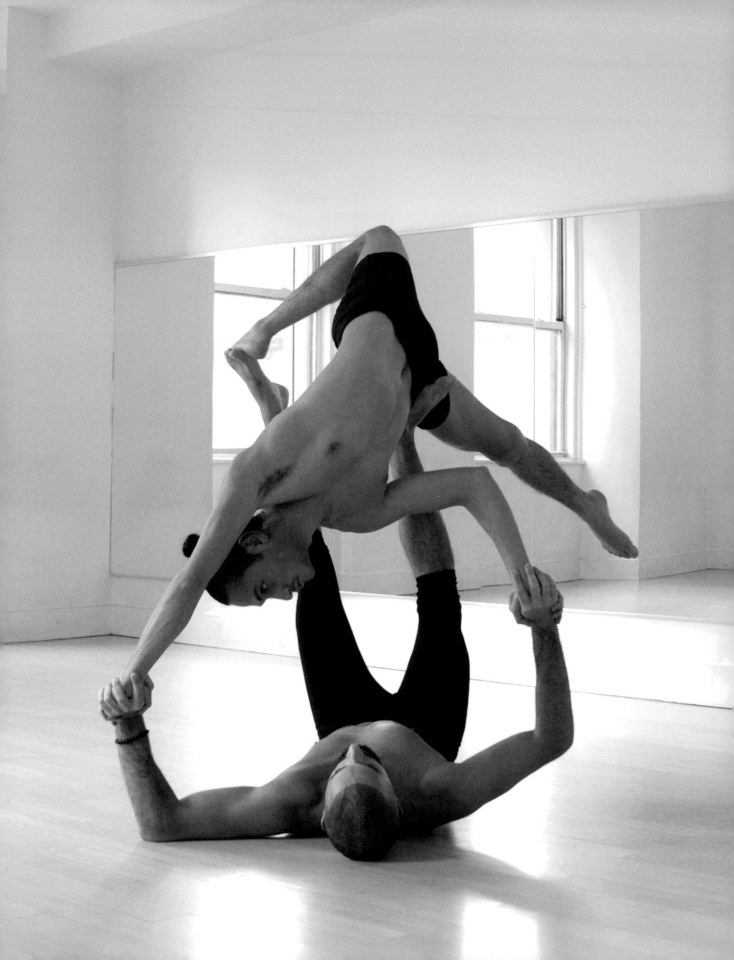

Nayef and Bassam

ACRO YOGA IMPROVISATION

• • •

Nayef (base position): I have not historically been an emotional person. I was born in America, but I am full-blooded Lebanese. Culturally, Middle Eastern men are taught to be emotionally disconnected. It's, "Hey, calm down; you're a man." I was uncomfortable showing *I am happy, I am angry*, or *I am sad*.

I also didn't like being touched. I don't know why, but a gesture like holding hands in public was massively uncomfortable. Yoga got me past that initial barrier of *it's OK to feel things*; then acro yoga, a blend of acrobatics and yoga, broke me through the touch barrier. Acro yoga isn't sexual, but it's extremely intimate, whether you're posing with men or women. It requires you to trust your partners. When I started doing it, all of a sudden I was OK with hugging in public.

Bassam (flying position): I came to the United States two years ago. I am from Iraq, but my family left in 2006 because of the obvious reason,

the invasion. It had become unsafe to live there. My dad said, "I'd rather spend money to have you guys live elsewhere, safe, than spend it as ransom after you get kidnapped and tortured." Now most of my family lives in Serbia.

In acro yoga, you're not always working with the same partners; you mix it up. I am moving from one pose to another on an unstable surface—another person. Fear sometimes kicks in. You're in a very vulnerable place, especially if you are trying a new pose. This forces you to form really strong relationships. You learn to trust lots of different people.

That's the power of the practice: it builds a community. When I came to the U.S., I knew absolutely no one. But after I took one acro yoga workshop, I had friends here. Now I consider them family. If I am traveling, two or three acro yogis will invite me to their houses. It is so great, so crazy. Everyone cares for everyone.

Mandy

STANDING HAND-TO-BIG-TOE POSE

• • •

I have learned everything I know about loving from teaching yoga, and in a way, I fall in love with each one of my students. When you practice with other people in the same room, you're literally breathing them in. I feel like with every person who has ever taken my class, there is a thread running from my heart to their heart forever. I often learn something about a student and never forget it.

Just to clarify, this kind of love is very different than romantic love. I choose not to date my students. I look at all of them as if they are my children. I know a lot of people love flirting, and it makes them feel really good, but I don't want to sexualize people who are practicing yoga. To me, that would make them feel unsafe.

Students do sometimes develop crushes on their teachers; it's sort of a natural thing that happens, but I believe it's a teacher's responsibility not to respond. I don't get crushes on my teachers—but if I did, I would not want to feel that they were attracted to me.

So if I'm talking with my students after class and I notice one of them seems to have developed feelings for me, I have this thing that I do. I put up a little invisible barrier and just keep moving.

That's because when I'm teaching people, I want to love them in a very neutral way. It's the universal love, the One Love—in Sanskrit, the *bhakti*. That's what everybody gets addicted to when they practice. Everyone wants that.

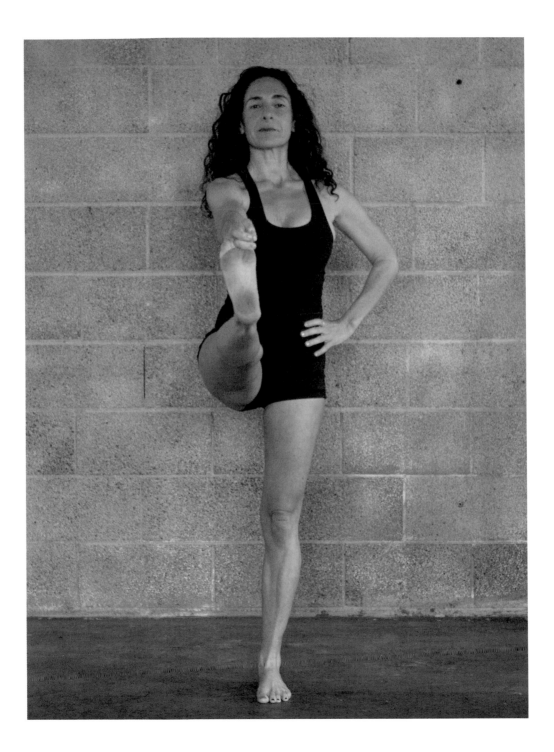

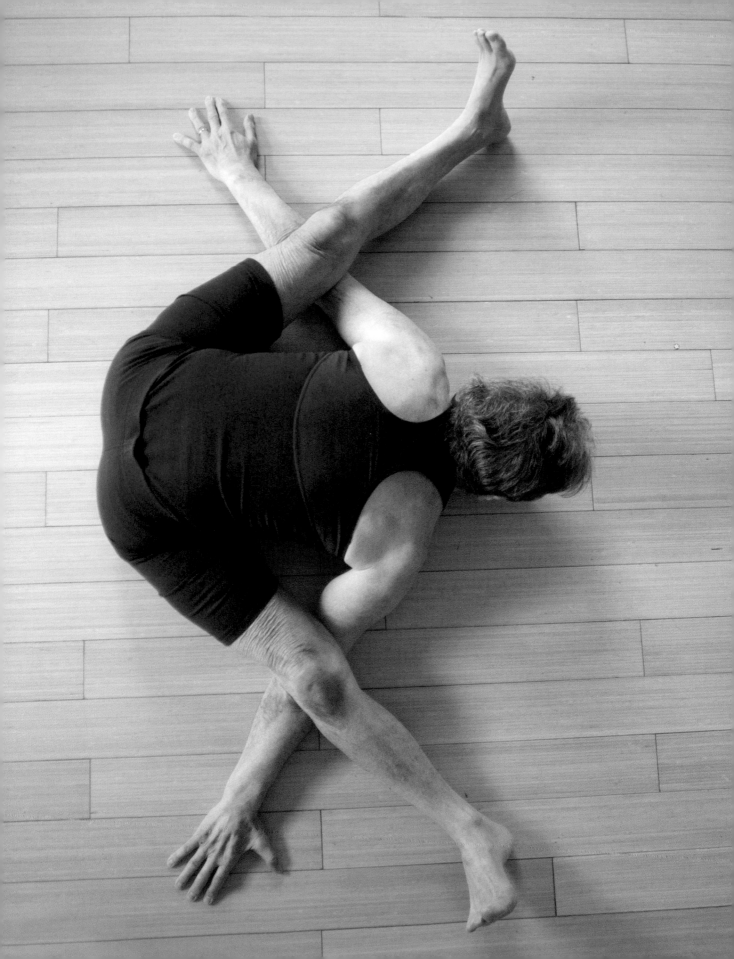

Loren

TORTOISE POSE

...

I was about nine years old and saw a movie—a version of *The Jungle Book*. There was a young boy in it who rode on the neck of an elephant and did something that resembled yoga. I said, "This is for me!"

Years later, my real introduction to yoga came when, as a graduate student in philosophy, I decided to go India and learn Sanskrit as part of my study of the origins of mathematics and grammar. I was there a few weeks when I realized I would never learn to use this ancient language the way a native Indian would. Instead, I wandered around India for about three years, had oodles of fun, and met many people who were seeking liberation and enlightenment far outside the bounds of academia.

During that time, I happened to meet an English drug addict in Bombay who handed me the book *Light on Yoga,* by B.K.S. Iyengar, one of the world's most influential teachers. I thought it was fascinating and resolved to do every pose in it (at least, that I was able to do) every morning and every night. After some time I sought out Mr. Iyengar and studied with him in Pune for a year.

Mr. Iyengar and I struck up a warm friendship—he was very generous and kind and intelligent—and at the end of the year, he said, "Don't stay here." He thought I should return home and share what I had learned, which was that yoga could be used to heal physical ailments.

So I did. Today, I am a doctor. I use yoga along with Western medical techniques to help patients in my physical medicine and rehabilitation practice, and I practice yoga myself every day.

I think the more yoga people do, the better. People often try yoga to help with physical problems, but I would like to see them get more enthusiastic about its mental benefits. It addresses so much of what matters. Not just the physical, but your relationship to other people, your relationship to the universe. That's what yoga is about.

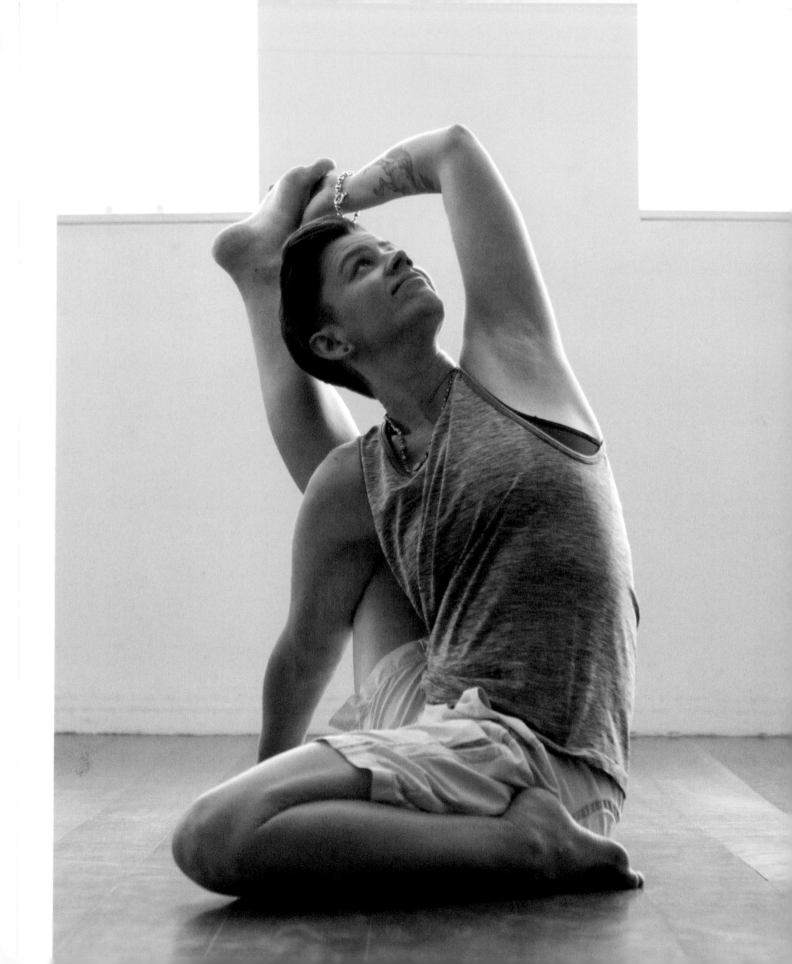

Miles

SUNDIAL POSE

· · ·

I don't feel super excited about the binaries of man/woman, male/female. I think of myself as a boi. That's the word if you have to use one, though I don't love labels, either. I'm not trying to be eccentric, just honest: There has been a little boy living in me ever since I was tiny.

In Colombia, where I grew up, very clear boundaries delineate what is "woman" and what is "man." Women look a certain way; they get their nails done; they're perfectly put together. I never felt like I fit in, but I played the role to get by. When you are like me, you live with a low—sometimes high—buzz of fear that some stranger will hate you for your in-betweenness.

And it's exhausting to fight for every single bit of understanding, even from those who know full well who you are. A few years ago, soon after I started going by Miles instead of Mila, my girlfriend at the time broke up with me. I really loved her. She said, "How could you do this to me?" I wasn't doing this "to her." I guess things got a little too real.

That's the stuff that really hurts: the rejections from people who deep down love you, but whose acceptance only goes so far.

But the more I'm able to allow the little boy some play space, the sweeter things are. Letting myself lean into my masculine side has allowed me to indulge my softer, more feminine side. It's the best of all possible worlds.

This play of opposites is very yogic. In yoga, the guru, or teacher, is seen as the mother. The same Hindu deity can appear as masculine, feminine, or androgynous. If you look at depictions of the gods Brahma, Vishnu, and Shiva, they're incredibly feminine.

I'm a musician, and just as tension makes guitar strings sing, the tension between my masculine and feminine extremes brings me to life. I'm not afraid of my in-betweenness anymore.

Heather

POSE OF THE SAGE VASISTHA

...

There's an astrologer online a lot of people look up to, and somebody told me recently, "My friend once saw him standing in front of a soda machine and kicking it." You hear that, and your heart is broken into pieces. People get really thrown off if they see one of their idols behaving like a human.

I know what it's like to idolize people. In my early years of yoga, the teachers who resonated with me were gods in my mind. I wanted to dress like them, think like them, be like them. Everything about them was so perfect: They'd walk into class and have the perfect thing to say. They did the practice perfectly.

Eventually I got to know them and could see little schisms or downfalls. I'd notice they had some issues or see them gossiping. My heart was shattered, but I did get over it. I have come to see my teachers as human but still feel they have something meaningful to teach me. A really important spiritual step is to see a person you've idealized fall from the throne and to still love them, but with clarity, not illusions.

Now I'm a teacher and have a sense sometimes that people idealize my life. That especially happens if you're living the kind of yoga/travel/retreat/beach life I've created for myself.

The whole idea of idealism becomes humorous when someone idealizes you. I am a completely normal, sassy, expressive woman. I am traveling and doing yoga and posting photos of myself, but as much as my life looks like an easy, everything-falls-into-place situation from the outside, I know my own backstory, my day-to-day humanness, and how much I'm working and striving. I'm experiencing myself from the inside, which is full of all sorts of self-judgments, insecurities, and comparisons—flaws anybody could have.

No matter who you are, even if you're the most beautiful, richest person in the world, you're still going to experience those feelings because you're human. The point of yoga is to develop compassion for yourself. That will help you develop compassion for others. Yoga builds self-esteem in a humble way, reminding us of our sameness, not our differences.

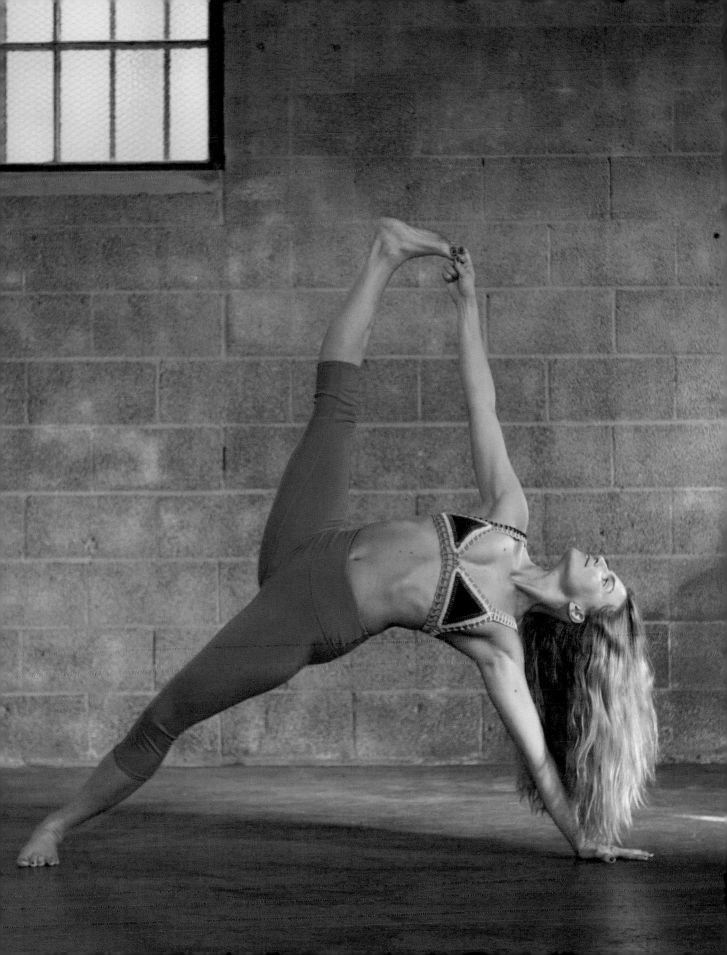

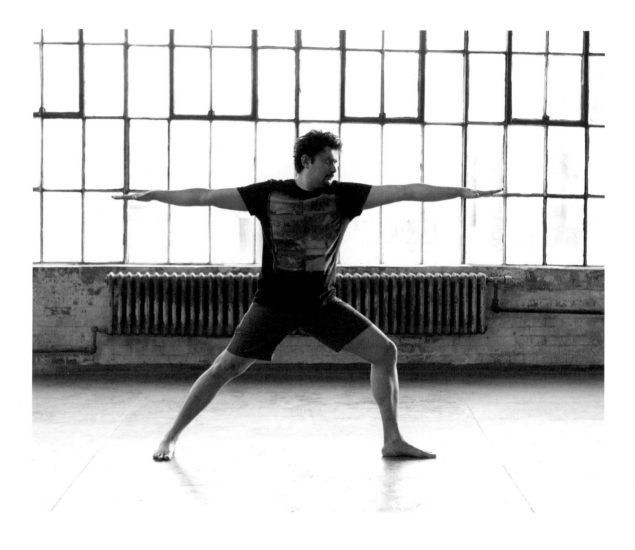

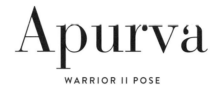

Apurva

WARRIOR II POSE

• • •

Yoga is about incrementally becoming more aware of the world around you and of yourself: your thoughts, decisions, and behaviors. When you start doing yoga, you begin thinking, "What are the consequences of my actions? Why am I doing what I am doing? Will it be beneficial to me? Are there negative implications?"

The main principle on which Hinduism is based is karma, the idea that our lives are defined by how we act and that everything we do has consequences, which can be good or bad. I would never tell anyone not to eat meat or drink alcohol, but I would recommend that anyone who wishes to eat meat consider the effect of that choice. That might mean going to see how animals are butchered and processed. Likewise, if you choose to drink, you might first go to a bar and observe people getting drunk.

Hindus believe that every single thing we do, every single thought, can affect our karma for the next seven generations. If you come from that awareness and see things from that perspective, you understand that your actions matter and everything in the universe is yours.

When you realize that you own everything, you start to take responsibility for everything.

Lauren

BOW POSE

...

I am incredibly bad at yoga. I am surprisingly bad. And I'm sort of past the point of trying to get better at it.

All of the things I'm bad at come together in yoga. I am uncoordinated. I have terrible balance. I have never been flexible. I can't touch my toes. I am bad at following directions for anything physical. If the teacher says, "Today we're going to do Gilded Unicorn Pose!" and then demonstrates how to do it, I'm the one standing around afterward watching everybody else because I can't remember the steps. I cannot count the ways in which I've been adjusted because I'm not doing something right.

When I walked into my first class fifteen years ago, you would have looked at me, a fit young woman, and thought, "Sure, she can do yoga." I assumed I would eventually be good at it. And at my peak, I was going to class four or five times a week, still under the impression that I was going to get better.

Now I have a full-time job, and children, and I can't get to yoga more than a few times a month. I'm not in good shape, and I'm exhausted. I can't do some poses I used to be able to get into.

But I've been surprised to realize that when you scrape away the ambition and superficial fitness element, you see yoga's true value in what remains. Yoga makes me so happy. I'm no longer impatient about it. I enjoy it more than I enjoy practically any other activity.

I still can't touch my toes. My hands get past my knees, but not to my feet. I was talking to a teacher the other day about this, and he said, "That is so amazing! You're *in the practice.*" It felt good to hear—that when I try to touch my toes, I'm in the moment, in the struggle. There's something profound happening there that wouldn't happen if I could do it with no effort.

There has to be something to that. Otherwise why would I keep bothering to practice an activity that by any other measure I stink at?

44

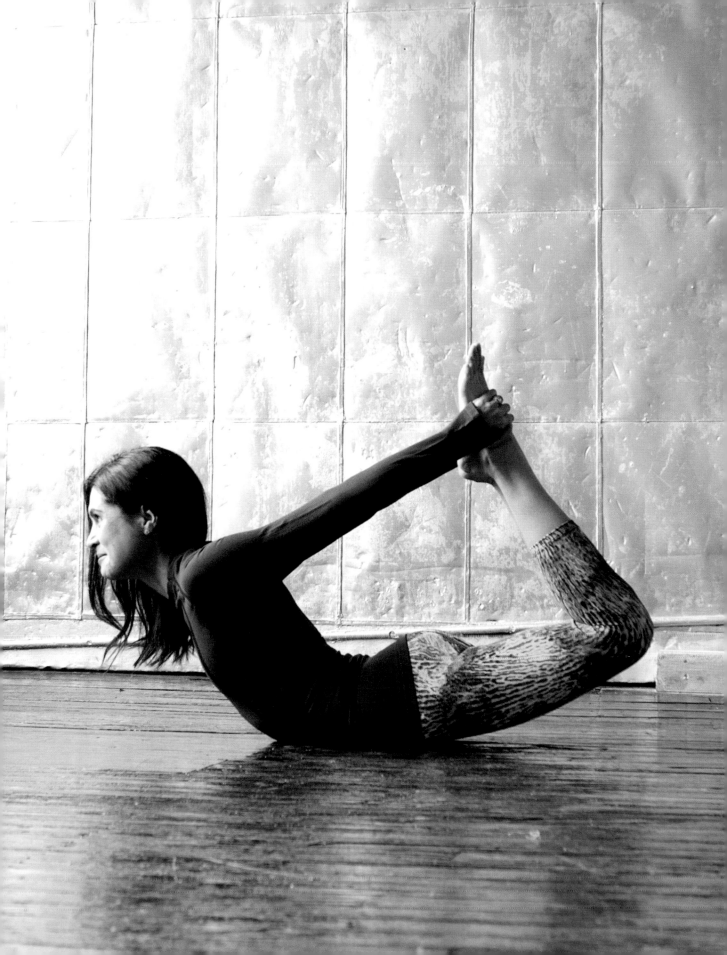

Dana

BIRD DRINKING RAINDROPS POSE

...

A lot of yoga teachers are former actors. One reason is that the art of acting is the art of being human, and yoga helps you rediscover the depth and the possibility of being human.

Acting is a very challenging business for a woman because you are held up to unreasonable standards, and often the way you look affects your income and your artistic fulfillment. I started practicing yoga regularly so that I would continue to look a certain way. I stayed with it because I found I could do challenging poses; but what really won in the end was the way yoga made me feel, which proved to be much more transformational than how I looked or what I could do.

I have played Julia in *The Two Gentlemen of Verona*, Olivia in *Twelfth Night*, and Beatrice in *Much Ado About Nothing*—sixteen Shakespeare plays over the course of my career. I miss the ensemble and working on a team, and I miss Shakespeare. But while acting itself is fantastic, competing for jobs can be dreadful. I lost parts for being too young, too old, too tall, too short, too ethnic, and not ethnic enough.

One time, during a callback, I overheard a casting director talking the director out of hiring me. He said, "Dana is like a cake that has frosting but no insides." I have been accused of a lot of things, but not having depth isn't one of them! I didn't get that part.

I haven't acted for a long time. Great jobs will come up, and I'll consider them reasonably and think, "Would I really rather do this instead of what I'm doing now?"

The answer is usually no; my work as a yoga therapist and yoga teacher is so satisfying and means so much to me.

And even though yoga itself is a competitive business, and there's a hustle to it, the worst day in yoga is never as horrible as a bad day in acting.

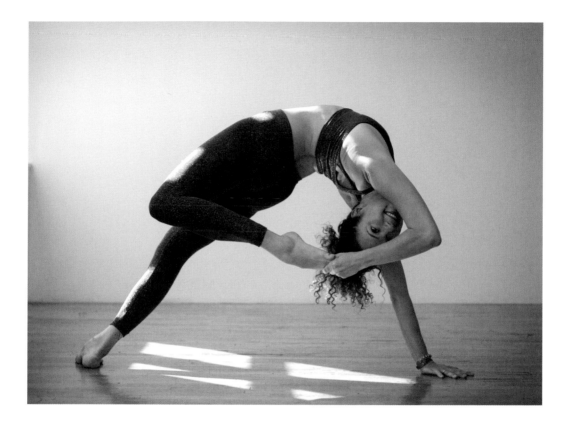

Rudra

SEATED LOCUST POSE

...

A yoga ashram is like a commune. It's group living for people who follow one particular spiritual teacher and who want to immerse themselves in their yoga practice. Most ashrams are kind of like a summer camp, in that any layperson who wants to can visit and learn about the teachings. Some people commit their life to the ashram and become a swami, which is a monk, or you can commit yourself to it for just a short period of time.

I am the manager of the Integral Yoga Institute ashram in New York City. Our building, which is connected to a yoga school that's open to the public, has twelve dorm rooms for people who live here full time, including me. I teach yoga, provide spiritual counseling as an ordained interfaith minister, and do administrative duties, and in exchange I get room and board and a clothing allowance; the other people pay a modest room and board. We practice

yoga together and have a meeting on Friday nights, and then the rest of the time we're out in the city working regular jobs. One guy here is a waiter, another is a financial advisor and yoga teacher, and one woman is a dance teacher.

When we have a space available, there are plenty of people who want to move in—these are affordable rooms in the middle of Greenwich Village, where rents are usually sky-high. I'm known as the gatekeeper, because it's my job to let people live here only if they really, really want to commit to the ashram lifestyle. If somebody expresses interest, I say, "Why don't you start coming to classes for a year and then talk to me again?" When you live in the ashram, you have to wake up every morning at six for meditation. When I first moved in, my initial thought was, "I could never do that," but now I'm doing it every day.

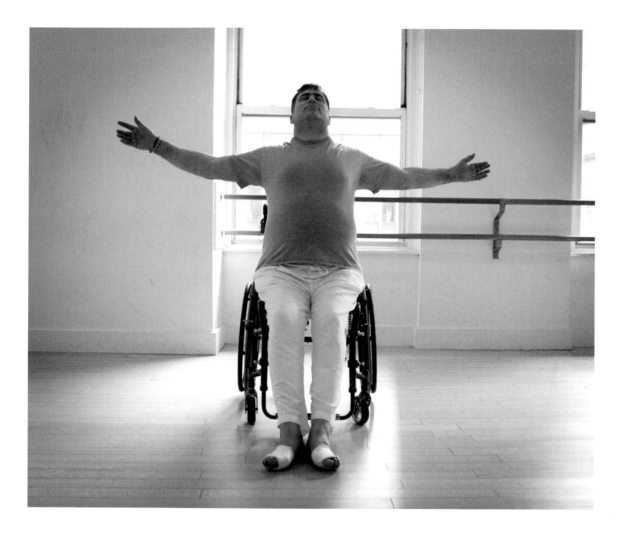

Zara

DRAGON POSE VARIATION

. . .

The first thing I gave up when I started doing yoga was junk food. I was in law school, living off of frozen corn dogs and macaroni and cheese out of a box, so the natural first change was to stop eating those things. I started to crave fruits and vegetables instead.

Next to go was the hard partying. By then, I was in a corporate-law job. This might surprise people who know me now, but I would stay out Friday nights until 6 a.m., drinking and doing lines of coke. I'd come home, take cold medicine to knock myself out for a couple of hours, and then get up and take a noon yoga class. That's a really unhealthy lifestyle. I knew it was unsustainable, so it was an easy one to let go of.

I also smoked tons of weed. I use to love to get high and then do yoga; I could get into deep stretches, and my balance was better.

But then I started attending Buddhist meditation retreats, and one day I opened up this box I had with a huge bag of weed in it and thought, "I don't even know how long I've had this." I asked my roommate, "Do you want my bong?" I didn't feel like smoking anymore. It killed my mental clarity.

I stopped eating mammals, and then chicken, for ethical reasons. Finally I stopped eating fish. I was at the grocery store one day and this Indian guy started talking to me. He said, "You take fish out of the water and they suffocate, so their last minute of life is complete anxiety. All of that nervous energy is released into their flesh, and then you eat it."

Eventually, I left my corporate job. On some days I do three hours of asana and other practices. I can't work a traditional office job, because I need that time. And I don't stay out late. If I do, I can't get up early to meditate.

Years ago, I read a teaching that said, "You'll know you're going deeper and deeper into yoga when it permeates all of your life." I've become more and more sure that yoga is one thing I'm committed to in this life. It dominates every part of my existence.

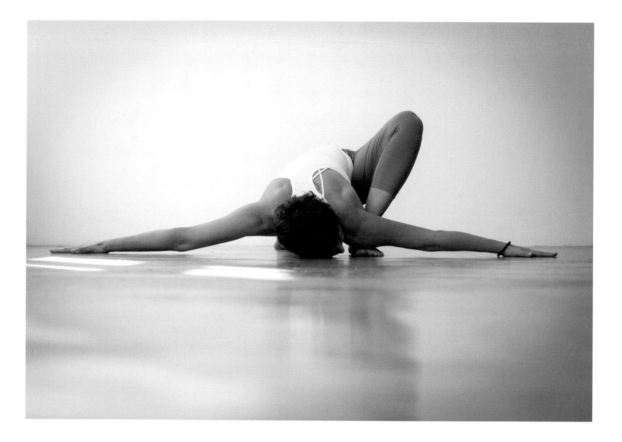

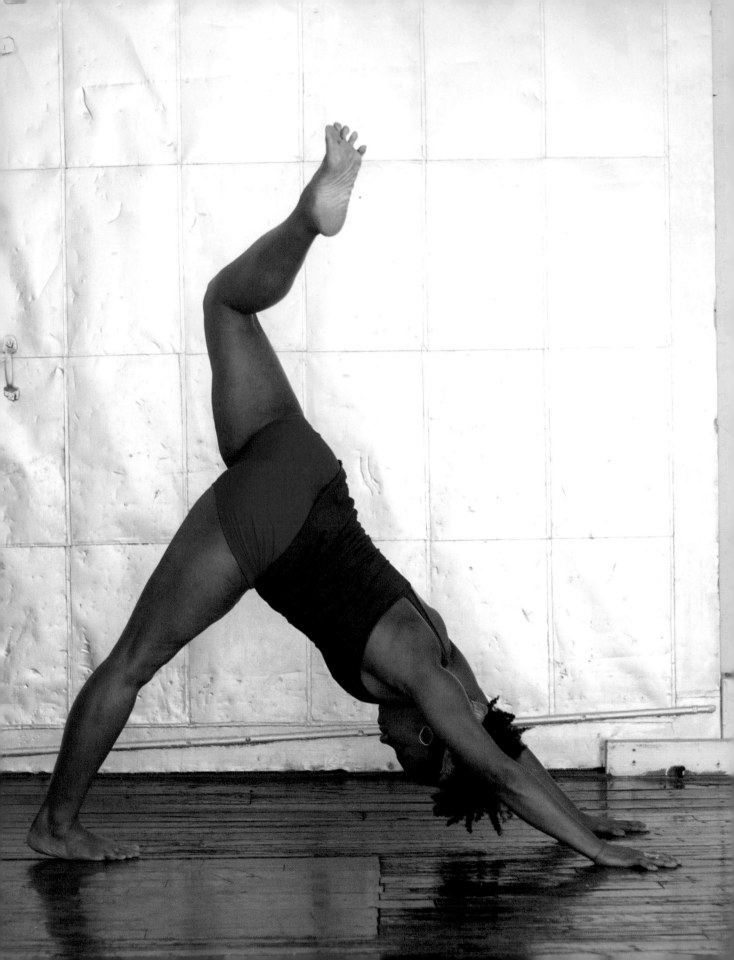

Crystal

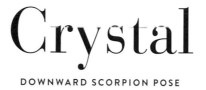

DOWNWARD SCORPION POSE

...

In the diverse population I work with, there are a lot of misperceptions about yoga. I have developed yoga programs for underserved urban schools and the Boys' Club of New York, and some of my little brown children have said things like, "Only white girls do that." When I tell them yoga comes from India and that it was once practiced only by brown-skinned men and boys, they don't always believe me. I have to make a case and present evidence.

For the adults, I spin it with a health-and-wellness bent. I talk about yoga as a tool that brings our body, mind, and heart into more balance so we feel better. Though the poses are only a small part of what yoga is, they're one way we access balance. When I tell people yoga can create more vitality and aliveness, they'll say, "I could use that." Everyone wants to be healthier.

In fairness, a lot of people have had negative experiences with yoga. They talk about going to a class and it was too hard, or they say they aren't flexible enough, or they describe feeling uncomfortable in a class with a lot of spiritual talk that seemed inauthentic to them. I say, "Listen, there are a zillion kinds of yoga. It sounds like the class you went to wasn't right for you." You can go to a great, sweaty flow class with music or try a more mystical, traditional style. Some styles always do the same sequence of poses; others vary the sequences. I definitely think it all has value.

In my own yoga practice, one thing I cherish is when teachers encourage me to think, experience, and make conclusions for myself. I once attended a yoga training seminar with a very famous teacher. I remember her saying, "To be a true yogi, you have to imbibe everything the guru tells you."

That was not how I was raised. I was raised and educated to think critically and be discerning. I thought, "I will take what you have to offer, but I will filter it through my truth meter." I believe a really good yoga teacher guides students to be their own guru.

Victor

DHARMA MITTRA HEADSTAND

· · ·

I learned about Buddhism in Catholic school. I remember my teacher saying in Global History class that Buddhism was a philosophy, not a religion, so you could be a Buddhist and still be a Catholic. This had an impact on me, because Buddhism was really resonating with everything I felt on a personal spiritual level. I thought, "This is kind of what I believe."

My coed school also had a yoga club, and a friend asked if I wanted to come. This was way before the yoga craze. Yoga was considered pretty out there and subversive. The only people who went to Yoga Club were, like, the weird people—a group I was proud to be a part of.

I was not the joyful person people know me to be today. I was fifteen and searching—for nothing specific, but nevertheless I was enveloped in my own sadness. I respected Catholicism and did not have any terrible experiences with it, but I was curious about yoga from a spiritual perspective.

Yoga Club met after school. We gathered in a classroom, pushed the desks aside and laid down our mats. Ten or fifteen people were there, including students, an art teacher, and a religion teacher. My Italian teacher, a Franciscan monk, led the class.

There was no inspirational discourse. The class was just Brother Ben leading us through very basic shapes. He would tell us how to get into a pose, and we would hold it. At the end was the final resting pose, Savasana. To this day, I remember coming out of the first yoga class of my life and feeling a radiant peace I had never felt before. There was no comprehension. There was no wondering. I wouldn't have been able to articulate it right then, but I knew, "This is it. This is how I want to feel."

No one has ever asked me what came up for me during that first class. Now that I'm talking about it, these poses unlock the body's energetic channels. I believe we're all born with karma, and that there was a lot of pain built up in me from previous lifetimes. I am not an enlightened being by any means, but in that first class I got a taste of what it felt like to be free.

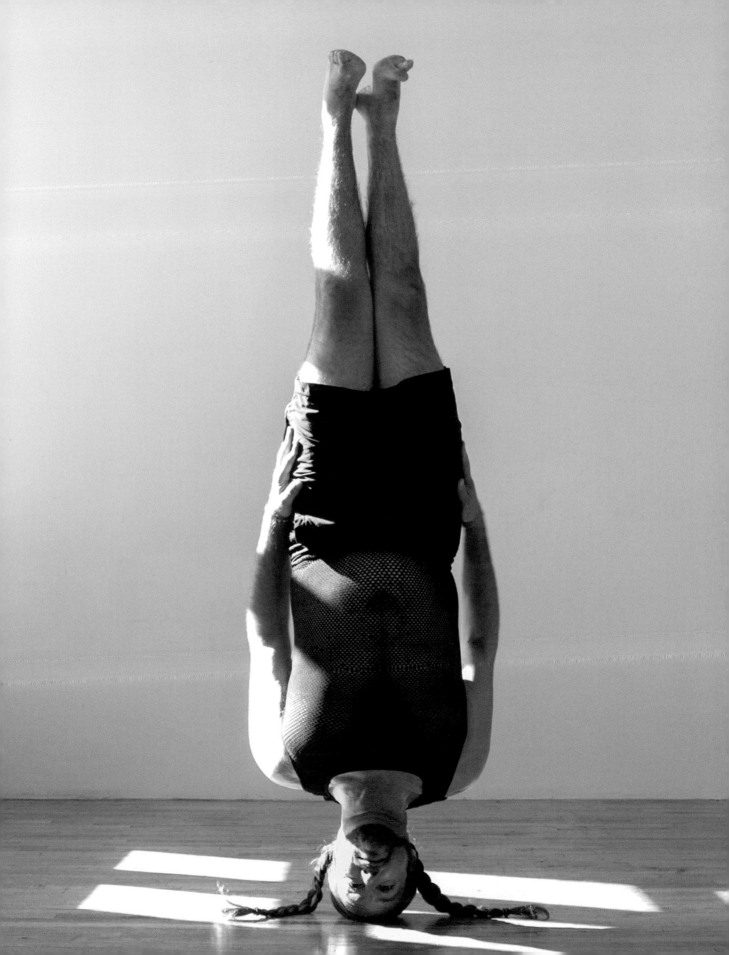

Halle

GODDESS POSE VARIATION

. . .

I had a student collapse once in a hot yoga class. I thought she was just being really elegant in her descent from her Talasana to her Uttanasana. Instead, she just kept folding forward and hit the floor. I was watching her and thinking, "Ah, that's so beautiful . . . oh, no, it's not! Woman down!"

Luckily, she didn't lose consciousness—nothing serious. But stuff like this happens, because hot yoga is gnarly. The first few times you try it, if you're not used to it, you're not in the moment, breathing. All you're thinking about is, "I am so friggin' hot!" When you teach hot yoga, you really have to make sure your students stay hydrated and drink, and I'm not talking about wine coolers.

I was scared, but I held it together. I went over to her to make sure she was OK. She was, and she wanted to stay, so I put her head in my lap and sat there with her and kept teaching. You are responsible for all of your students' well-being in a class. When one of them has trouble, you take care of them, but you still have to keep the space for everyone else there.

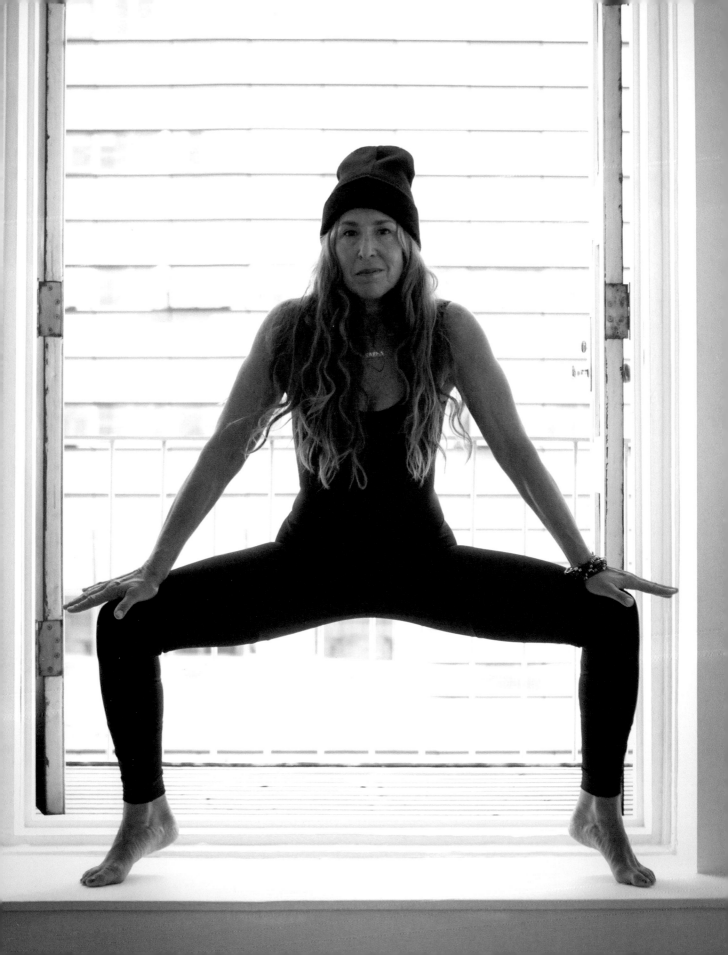

Maezen

STANDING SIDE BEND

...

I love to do yoga with a mirror. Some people don't like it, but I find the mirror is a marvelous tool that allows me to balance and center myself. If the mirror disturbs me, that is a sign that I might need to focus my practice on recognizing the degree to which I am still involved with my ego.

If you are judgmental, if you take an egocentric view of yourself—and by "egocentric" I don't mean arrogant, but just very self-conscious—then the mirror will be a distraction.

We tend to be critical when we're comparing ourselves to others: "She's so skinny. Why can't I look like her?" or "Look at him. He's doing it wrong." But yoga starts with your relationship with yourself. We're there on our mats to cultivate a single-pointed concentration. So the mirror doesn't distract me. And, practically speaking, I find it easier to do balancing poses when I look into a mirror and gaze into my own eyes. It gives me something to focus on.

There may be a lot of people who practice yoga with a mirror for the purpose of admiring themselves. But that's the opposite of what a spiritual practice is.

As a Zen Buddhist priest, I have found that ultimately the signpost of maturity in any practice is humility and selflessness. The more you do it, the more completely disinterested you are in yourself.

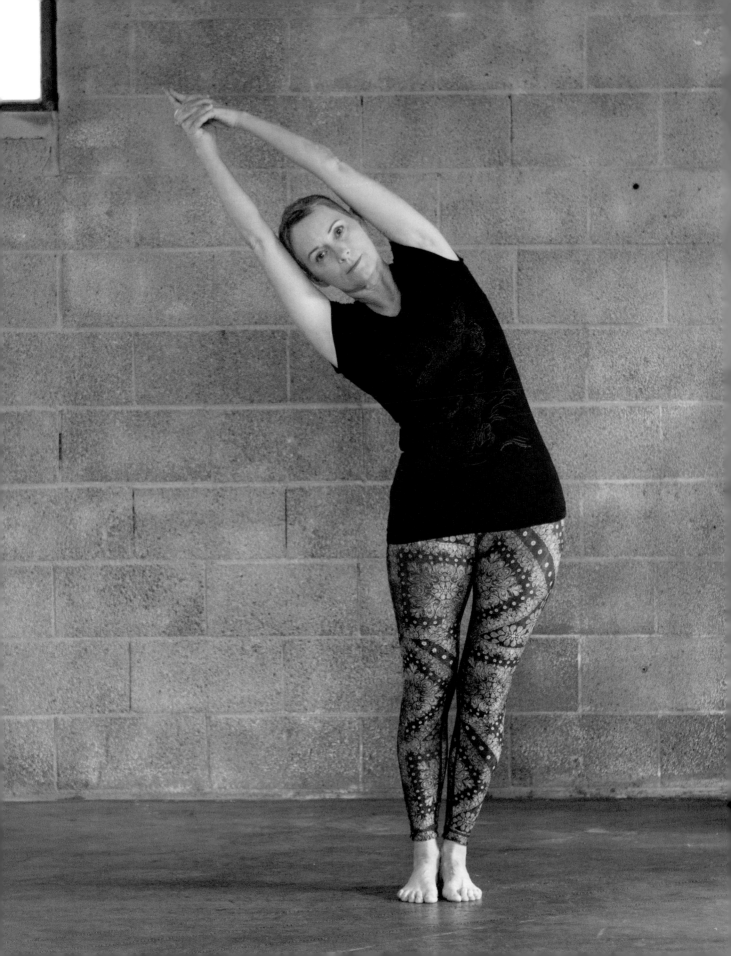

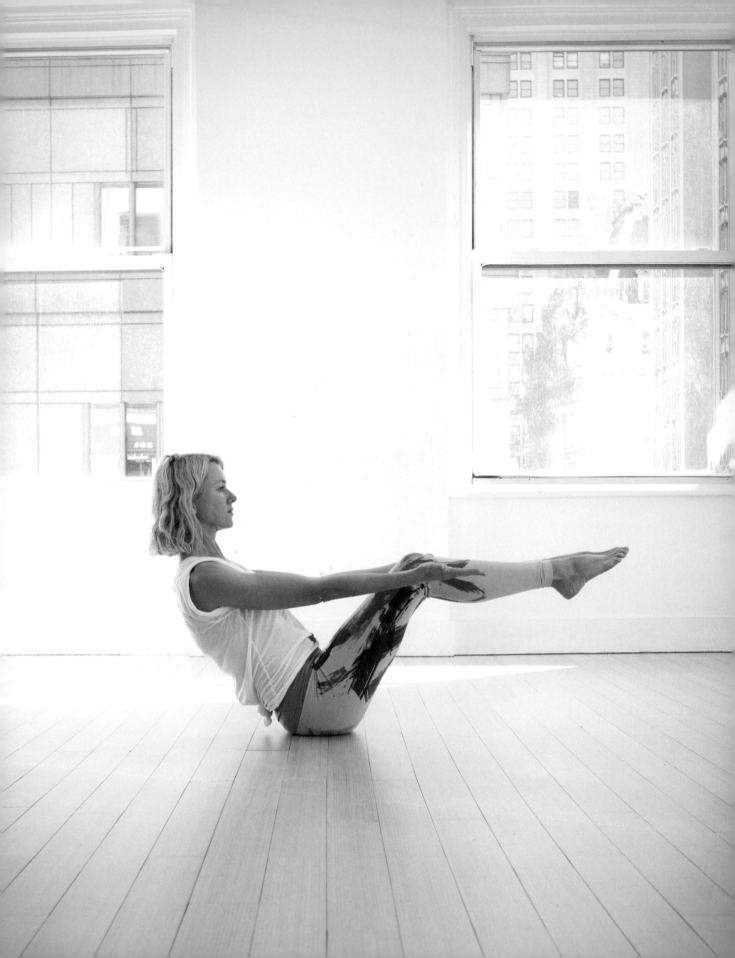

Naomi

...

I have been practicing Ashtanga yoga for twenty years. It is a pretty strenuous form of yoga that is very challenging but also rewarding. I even got to practice for a week in New York many years ago with the late Pattabhi Jois, who was the founder of Ashtanga. I was filming night shoots at the time; I remember I would go straight from the set in the morning to the studio, just to be in his presence.

It was an incredibly powerful experience. I could do poses that I hadn't previously been able to do and haven't done since.

Now as I'm getting older I can feel my body changing. I don't approach yoga the same way anymore. I concentrate on stretching and healing, and on helping with circulation and mindfulness. I'm more gentle and don't push myself beyond my body's limitations. I sometimes have back issues, so I don't jump from one pose into another anymore.

I try to separate my body and my ego. That's easier to do at this stage in my life and leaves me feeling energized and fulfilled.

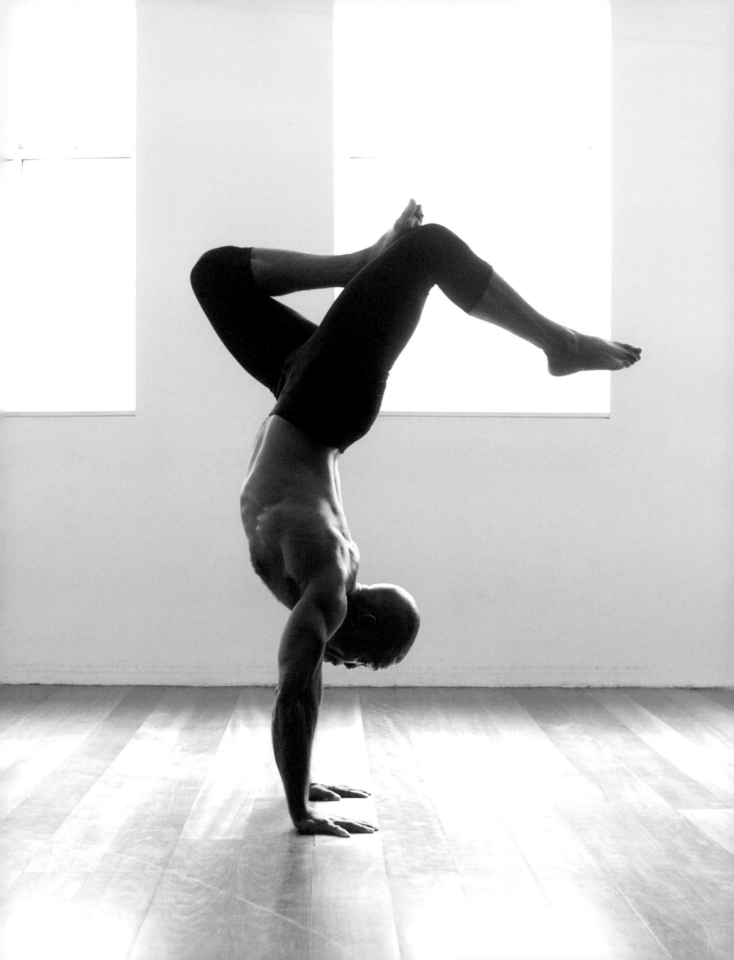

Esco

HALF-SCORPION VARIATION

· · ·

I got into fitness during a very difficult time in my life. Working out offers a pathway to a certain level of ease in your mind, a certain level of control in your thoughts. But yoga literally changed me. I went in with one philosophical view and came out different.

When I was eighteen, I made a decision that I wanted to be a drug dealer. It went OK for about a year, until I got caught and did three months in jail.

That didn't discourage me. Instead, while I was in County, I decided that I didn't want to be a drug dealer—I wanted to be a *superhero* drug dealer. I justified it by telling myself that the criminal conviction had left me with no other options in life.

At the time, I was attending college. I didn't sell to students, and they didn't know anything about me. They saw me as the president of the Paul Robeson Club, a person with good grades. I threw all the parties and drove a nice car. People said,

"How the hell do you have that Lexus?" I was like the fake Puff Daddy of Rutgers University.

I actually loved school. I got a degree in business management and then started on a master's. I dropped out of graduate school with just one final paper to write because my business had really started growing. I was selling cocaine and crack to suburban middle-class Caucasian, Latino, and black people in New Jersey, Pennsylvania, and Ohio. I wouldn't touch it—not cocaine; hell, no. But it didn't bother me that other people were being harmed.

Then, in 2001, a cop pulled me over and found a brick of cocaine in the trunk. This time, I was going to federal prison.

Why did I choose the path of selling drugs? Well, all of my friends in high school were engaged in it at some level. I wasn't completely scared of it. And when you are young, you ask yourself, "How am I going to win the game of life?" You can say, "I'm going to be in the Army."

CONTINUED NEXT PAGE

"I'm going to play sports." "I'm going to work my way up the food chain." I figured I could never have a professional, white-collar career, but I could learn everything about business and be an entrepreneur.

I also did it to pay for school. That was my justification. I was young, and it was stupid and a very bad decision and insensitive. No one can afford college, yet people still find ways to pay for it that don't include selling drugs.

But after my second arrest, it was over. I told everyone in that world, "I quit." I cut off everybody. Now I have zero interest in selling drugs. The idea is nauseating.

Before I went to prison, I went home to spend a month with my father and little sisters. I wanted to write my final paper and get my master's degree. Ten days after I got to prison, my diploma arrived in the mail.

I spent forty-eight months in prison at Fort Dix, New Jersey. I was not a violent criminal, so this was a minimum-security facility. I felt anxiety early on, but I was able to man up and handle it. I had done this to myself; it's not like somebody did me wrong.

But I knew I was going to have to do jail a certain way. While I was there, I read and studied urban economics for hours a day. At the same time I was like, "OK, I need a job."

In prison, everyone works out, and people liked to work out with me. I met another inmate, a physical therapist serving time for insurance fraud who had started a kind of gladiator school in the prison, where inmates could learn how to be personal trainers. I thought, "I'll give that a shot." A lot of guys coming out of prison were the best personal trainers. They'd motivate people and make them work harder by, like, making fun of them. I decided, "If I'm going to do this, I'm going to be a mastermind at it."

I trained with that program for eight hours a day. If there's a way to be successful in prison, I was very successful.

I got out and was hired by a health club. I became the number-one trainer in the whole company. I was running small group fitness classes and looking for ways to bring in new clients. By then I was taking hot yoga once a week and decided to get formal training as a yoga instructor and use it to create a feeder program at my club. I thought, "People will take my yoga class, and they will say, 'You're amazing,' and I'll say, 'Thank you. Now come take small group training.'"

But the whole teacher training was an epiphany. It was ten-hour days and reading the *Bhagavad Gita* and sitting with my mentor. When I was done, I didn't care anymore about the feeder program. It wasn't, "I'm going to use yoga to build my other business," it was, "I'm going to help people train their minds, and that's going to give them peace."

I still have ambition. I am still a risk taker. But I avoid certain types of energy. I've stopped hanging around certain types of people. I've made a decision to practice yoga every day.

I don't go to the hot room for a workout; I'm there to find myself. To find my breath. To meditate in every pose.

It helps me feel like a superhero, to be honest. Seriously, that's how I feel.

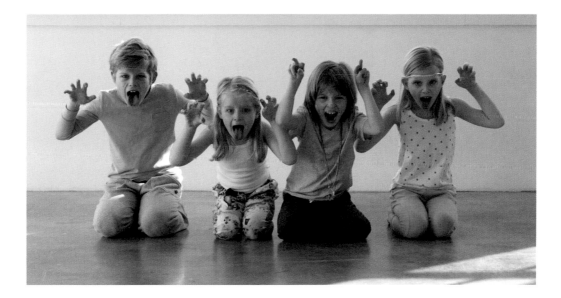

Loch, Olive, Gus, and Blake

LION POSE

• • •

Loch: Lion Pose is claws, tongue out, and angry-looking eyes. You're less mad when you're done 'cause of the eyes. Doing those eyes kind of makes you angry, and when you stop, that gets all of the mad out of you.

Oliver: I felt like a lion

Gus: I was really just doing a lion face. I'm not sure what I was thinking.

Blake: It made me feel like one of the guys from KISS.

Heather

CROW POSE

...

I was in a yoga workshop when my phone started vibrating. I could hear it from my mat. It was a new phone; I had just gotten it the day before and didn't know how to turn it all the way off. In a moment of panic, I went over to my bag and tried to bury the phone more deeply in case it vibrated again. When someone's phone goes off in class, it drives the other students crazy, which is why nobody ever admits when it's theirs.

When I teach yoga, I strongly discourage people from bringing their phones into the studio. If I see someone on their mat texting before we start, I'll ask them to step out until they're done. Because if they've left work, found a babysitter for their kids, decided not to go to the grocery store instead—if they've gone to all of that effort to come to yoga, then I encourage them to follow through and really let go of their obligations while they're on the mat. "Let this be your time," I tell them. Among other things, this means unplugging.

But sitting with yourself without the easy distraction a device provides—people have a very difficult time doing that. Without distractions, stuff comes up. And I don't mean nagging thoughts like, "I need to go the grocery store." I mean all of the stuff you've managed to avoid: the uncomfortable thoughts, the relationships that didn't work out, the bad feelings you've had about yourself. If you always have a device in front of you, you never need to confront those things.

I would never forbid a student from bringing a phone into the studio, but if I could, I would ask everyone to turn their devices off and put them away not just at the beginning of class but a few minutes before class, to help them transition into their practice. I don't know if that's a realistic request. Devices are so much a part of our culture now.

But I try not to sweat the small stuff, honestly. If your phone rings in class, your phone rings in class. It's not the end of the world.

68

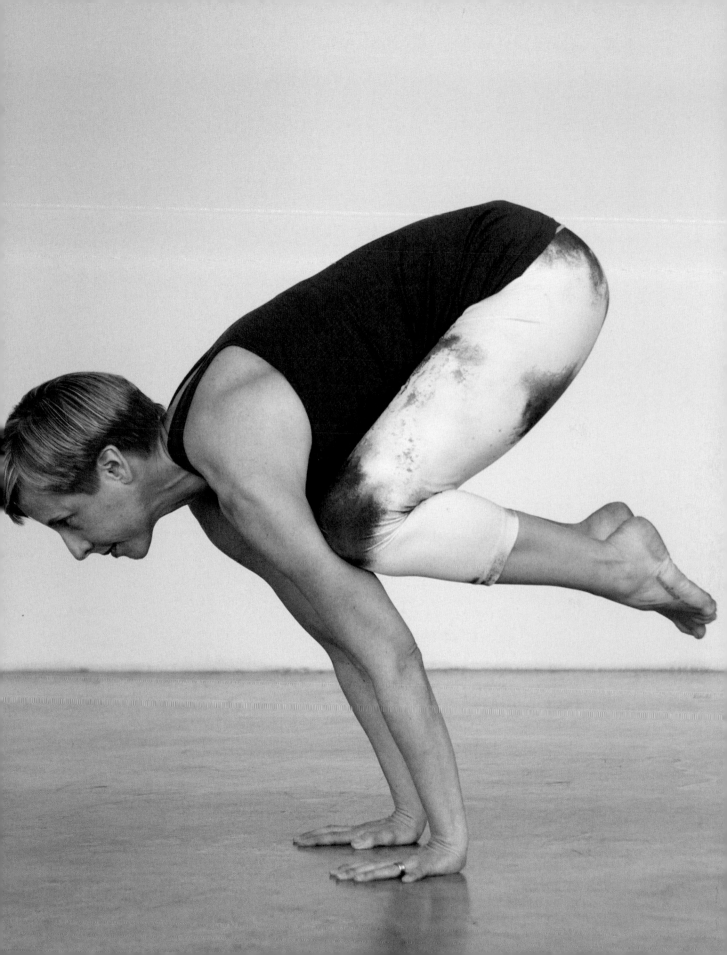

Michelle

EXTENDED HAND-TO-BIG-TOE POSE
AND
COBRA POSE (NEXT PAGE)

• • •

Last year I was in a very dark place. I lost my aunt, who'd been like a mother to me after my own mother died a few years ago. You think your parents are going to take care of you and make you feel better, no matter how old you get. That's what I lost. And then I really lost myself.

My husband is great. I love him, and he is always there for me. But after my aunt died a part of me was just gone. I felt unlovable, and I used food to numb the pain. We all know what chocolate does: I'd think, "OK, I'm going to eat this sugary thing, and for a little while, at least, I'll feel better." But as with any addiction, it was only a quick fix. I was in a cycle of overindulging.

Then I saw a video online of a military veteran, a paratrooper who had damaged himself from all of the jumps he did and was told he would never walk without braces. He had overcome his disability through a style of yoga called DDP. I watched how hard he'd worked to gain his life back. I said, "If he can do it, I can do it. I need to find that strength inside myself again."

I was telling this story to a cousin, and she said, "My friend Jesse just got his DDP instructor certificate. I'll ask him to get in touch with you." The next day, Jesse messaged me and encouraged me to try the program.

At first, I ordered DVDs and did them at home. I was too embarrassed to go to a studio, so Jesse coached me with online messages. I was so down on myself. When I'd say, "Oh, I am so fat," he would say, "We're going to work on that." He gave me my motto: One meal, one workout, one day at a time. When you're in a depression, just getting through daily life seems monumental and overwhelming. He would say, "Go do one workout. It's only twenty minutes. Just go do it."

After about a month, Jesse convinced me that I was ready to come into the studio. He had a friend, Chris, who was training as a DDP instructor and needed to practice teaching a student. That's how Jesse got me in, by persuading me to help his friend. When I walked into the studio, Chris showed me old pictures of himself to help me

CONTINUED NEXT PAGE

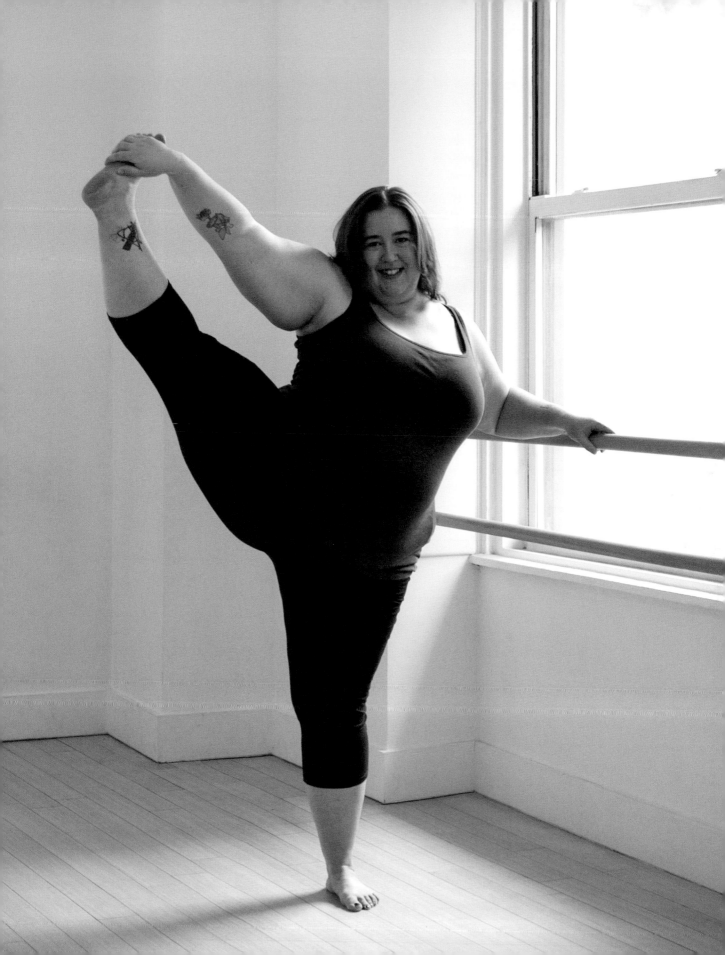

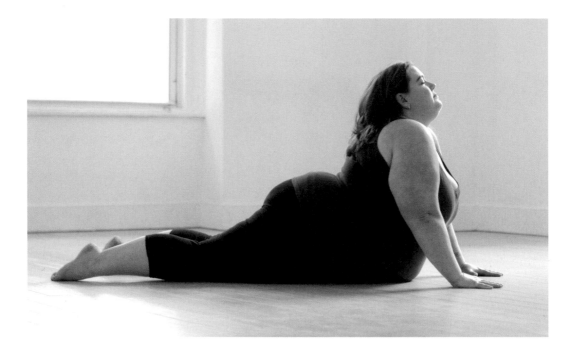

feel more comfortable. He said, "Look, this is me." He used to weigh three hundred pounds. I felt like I was around other people who understood my struggles.

Now Jesse, Chris, and I support each other. We're like the ragtag band of misfits. Jesse took a video of my first workout, and now, whenever I think about how far I have to go, I can look back and see how far I've come. At first I had to hobble down the studio stairs. I couldn't do certain poses because they hurt my knees. I couldn't get up off the floor without help.

Change is scary because you don't know what you're going to find. Looking at myself in a mirror and saying, "I love my body the way I am now, not for the way I should be"—that's also hard, because we live in a society where we're told we have to look a certain way to be lovable.

For me, it's a constant, daily effort. When I see somebody skinnier than me, or more beautiful, I say, "That's OK. She's on her own path. I'm lovable because I'm here."

As I look at myself doing these poses, I am proud.

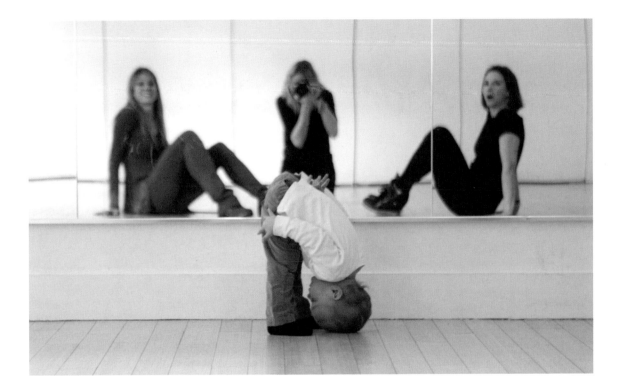

Shane

STANDING FORWARD BEND

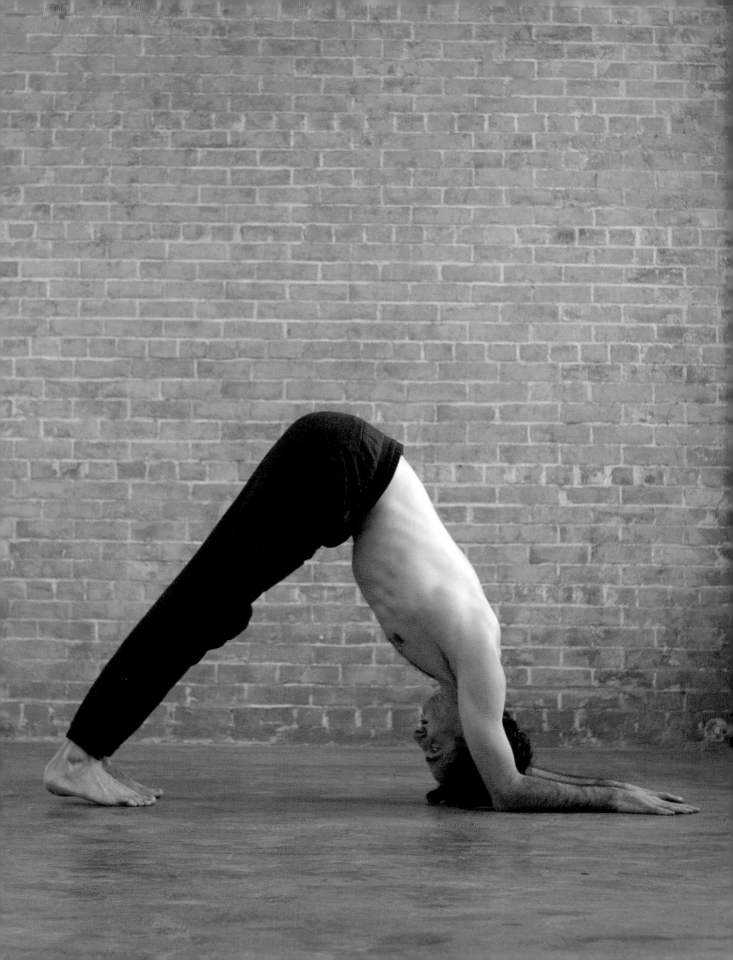

Josh

DOLPHIN POSE

. . .

The first few years out of a PhD and into a teaching job are hectic, because you're learning to teach and putting together your courses. In addition to that, I am also organizing a symposium, and then there's my biggest preoccupation: getting my book together. Publishing a book is the only way I will be able to keep my job. To become a tenured professor you have pull out all of the stops.

I have been practicing yoga since I was nineteen and in college. I grew up skiing, which brought on some lower-back pain, and yoga helped me with that. The practice also helped me cultivate a space separate from all of the striving and intellectual focus of the rest of my life. I need yoga to feel good physically, and I need it to maintain my equilibrium, psychologically and emotionally.

Part of the real lesson for me in a yoga class is learning to benefit from the collective group energy in the room, to resist the urge to compete, and to shed the conventional idea of achievement. You have to be competitive to succeed at a competitive job. But yoga reminds us to be less focused on ourselves as individuals.

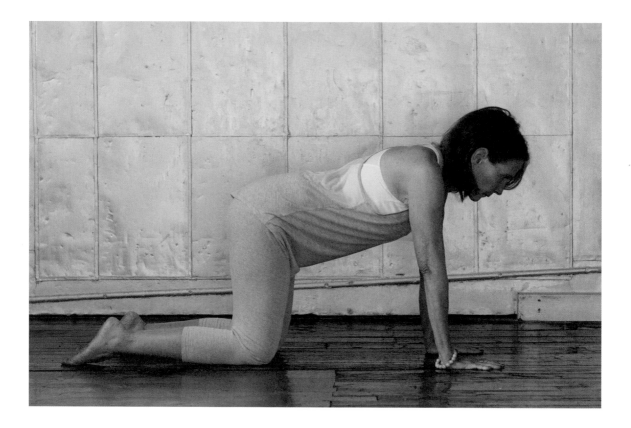

Angela

TABLETOP POSE

• • •

In your sixties, you're on a cusp. You start confronting your mortality and thinking, "What will happen to me ten years from now?" Your bones get weaker; there are balance and flexibility issues. I see hunched-over older people on the street and think, "I do not want to look like that." I don't want to be afraid to go outside because I might fall on a crack in the sidewalk.

My whole life, I exercised off and on—more off than on. I had fitness equipment in my tiny apartment. I went to gyms. But I was very unmotivated, even though I knew that exercise should be a priority. I would say, "Nah, I don't feel like it today. I'm too tired."

Eventually, though, I could no longer deny that I needed to boost my strength to fend off all of those horrible things older people fear.

I'd always had the idea that yoga was for twenty- or thirtysomething women. I didn't think it was for me. But after I started going to senior centers to pursue other interests, like opera, I noticed that most of these places teach some form of yoga. Also, I have a childhood friend exactly my age who has been doing yoga all her life, and I see how she looks; I see how she feels. I really had to say to myself, "What are you waiting for? What excuse do you have?"

I have to say, far from dreading yoga, I look forward to it. I go three or four times a week and am disappointed if for some reason I can't get to class. I really enjoy the positions and the stretching. At the end of a class I feel better than I did when I started, so of course I want to do it again.

My classes also have become a community of other older women, some of whom I have befriended. Yoga is joyful.

Older people can do yoga. It can be done. It's never too late, seriously. It is really never too late.

Taryn

REVOLVED STANDING FORWARD BEND

. . .

I have always been very hard on myself. I grew up with an internal voice that constantly questioned my own worth. The day-to-day information I received from my friends and other people was so much the complete opposite of what that voice told me that eventually I started to think, "Either everyone is just trying to make me feel better, or there is something wrong with the way I see myself." When did I realize this? I don't know—three days ago? Really, it's still a work in progress.

I am a fiery person who has a lot of emotion I want to move out of my body, and yoga was one of the first things that helped lead me to a place of release. Yoga was my first experience of using my body while controlling my breath, connecting the two into what felt like a moving meditation. That was a mind-boggling discovery, and I loved the feeling. But soon I found that yoga, which draws you inward and gets you really quiet, wasn't enough. I need to pound the floor a little bit.

About six years ago, I had just had a baby and I started teaching a couple of the other moms in my building this new style of movement I had created, which I now call "the class." In the class, we work one muscle group at a time until we completely exhaust it. I like to say that once we've crushed the physical body enough, that's when we're "in." We're into the parts of ourselves that are not so loaded with other people's ideas, and we're feeling things we don't want to feel, like, "I'm not good enough." What I am trying to do is heal something that's inside of me, to feel these feelings so I can face them. It seems like lots of people need the same thing.

I try to make people aware of what they're saying to themselves. Then we use cardiovascular movements like shaking and jumping jacks to flush that negative energy out of the body. I also encourage people to yell. Sometimes they cry. It's a cathartic experience.

We end in silence, the same way a yoga session ends. I just think sometimes you have to get really loud to get really quiet.

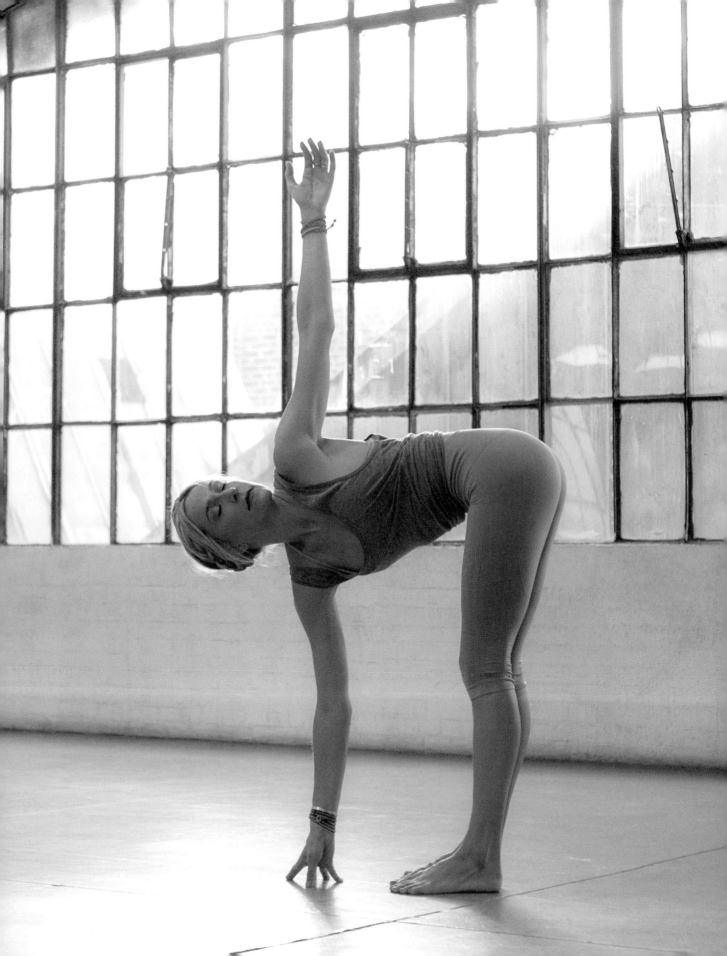

Arvind

SHOULDERSTAND

. . .

I got interested in yoga when I was probably fifteen years old and spending a couple of days visiting my uncle, who was a lawyer and a very good man. It was early in the morning, when I was partly sleeping and partly awake, that I saw my uncle doing yoga. I saw, *Oh, it's my uncle, standing on his head.*

I grew up in Mumbai, which was "Bombay" then. When I was first trying to learn yoga, I would go to a kind of exercise school, like a gym, near my house. In the courtyard, there was a wooden pole planted in the ground, and we used to try to hold the pole with two hands and raise up both of our feet. This was separate from meditation or anything like that. It was just a physical exercise.

I came to the United States in 1971. By then I was already done with medical school, and I was married. Originally I thought I would come here for a few years and learn some things, but then somehow one thing happened, and another thing, and we continued to stay. I practiced obstetrics and gynecology; our two daughters were born here, and the Indian population was increasing in our neighborhood, so we had comfortable surroundings.

I use yoga and meditation for peace of mind, and to relieve the stresses of life. As soon as a child is born, they get stress—they cry, right? So stress always comes to us. Yoga positions and meditation are a very nice way of relaxing. They keep our blood pressure down and our mind much more calm.

I used to be able to do the headstand, but I haven't done it for a while; I stopped when I began to get neck pain. I do Shoulderstand instead, which is a bit less strenuous. But I have been thinking: I am going to visit India in a few months, and I might try the headstand again.

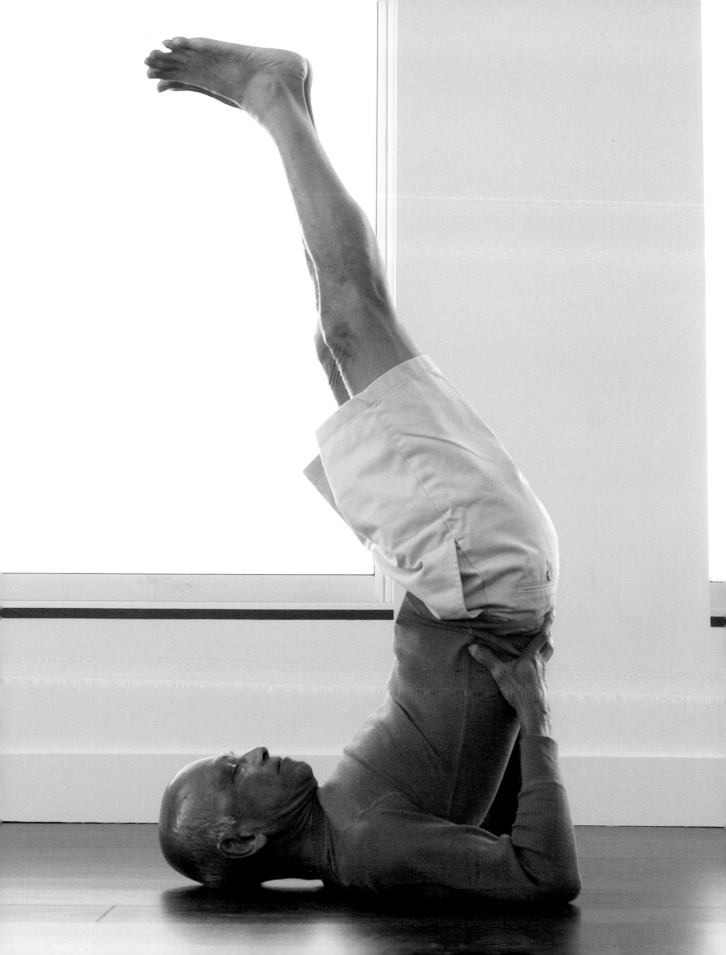

Adesuwa and Esosa

PARTNER BOAT POSE

•••

Adesuwa: It's so funny, because I had been trying to convince her to take yoga for years. I kept telling her, "Breathing and moving slowly can be liberating," and now she's repeating what I say.

Esosa: I like workouts that get my heart racing. I didn't think yoga would give me enough of a challenge. But I love my sister, and my sister loves yoga, so I jumped right into advanced classes. Frankly, I didn't get it. Yoga really, really wasn't my thing.

Adesuwa: It had taken me a while to get into yoga, too. When I first started, I went the same route as my sister later did: I took intense classes and didn't like them. I hate to work out; I'm the laziest thing ever. So I decided I would try a more mellow style.

A thirty-day yoga challenge I found on the Internet changed everything. I started following along with the online tutorials and enjoyed them; I felt like I was expressing myself and in tune with my body. The first time I did Downward Dog, my heels didn't touch the ground the way they're supposed to, but by the end of the thirty days,

though I didn't think I had worked that hard, my heels were down.

Yoga is a lot like life: At the beginning, you're not that good at it, but the more you do it, the better you are. That's what I was trying to explain to Esosa, but she kept saying, "I just don't like yoga. It really isn't for me."

Esosa: Then, only a few weeks ago, I had been doing these really intense weight workouts with a trainer, and I was so stiff and sore I could barely move. I thought yoga would kind of balance everything out. I remembered all of the things my sister had said and thought, "This time, I'll take her advice."

I took a basic introductory class. We were breathing and learning simple postures, and at the end I had almost a natural high. It was awesome. I was like, "Oh, all right; I get it."

Without taking the baby steps, I wasn't getting the best experience. Now I understand why everyone loves yoga so much.

Adesuwa: I'm laughing. This is what I kept telling her.

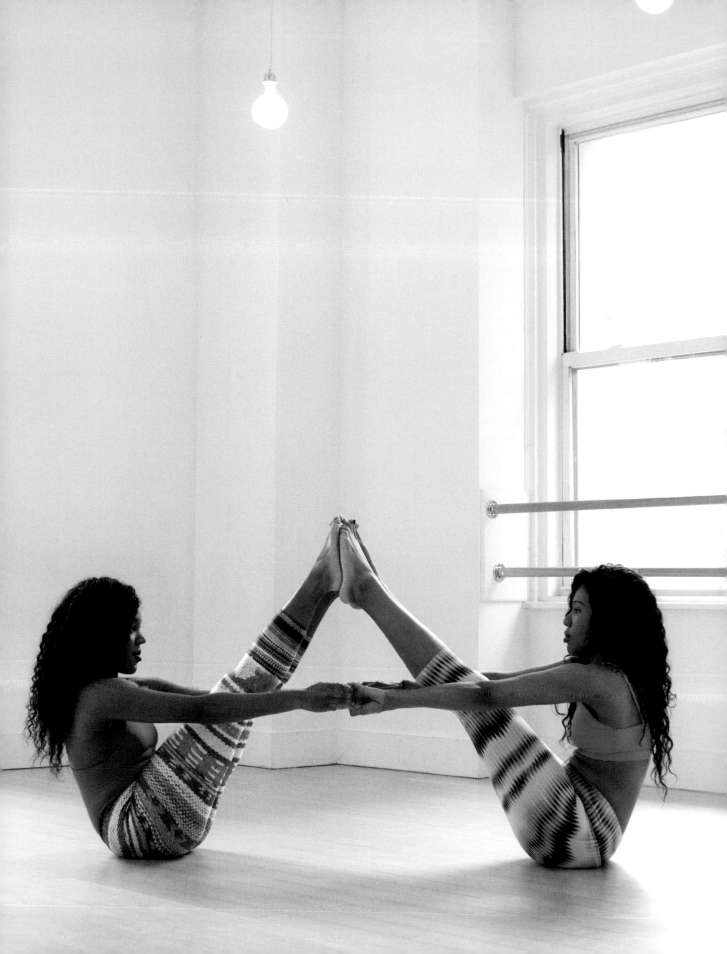

Claudia

HAPPY BABY POSE

...

I don't like yoga. I'm the editor of a sports and fitness website and probably shouldn't admit this, but I have to make myself do yoga. There are things we do because we like them—I love paddling, running, and skiing—and then there are things we have to do to improve our wellness and flexibility. For me, yoga is in that second category.

Why don't I like it? To begin with, I don't get why we have to listen to New Age music in class. It's clichéd. I don't find it relaxing. I find it irritating.

Another thing that drives me crazy is that the teachers don't demonstrate. They'll say, "Put your left leg by your right toe and lift your left knee," and I'm like, "What?" I spend half the time peeking under my arm at the person next to me to see what I'm supposed to be doing.

In fact, yoga overall isn't a Zen experience for me. You go into a studio and they pack you in. People always come late—I don't know why that's OK; it's a weird code of yoga behavior—so even when you've sort of found your spot,

you have to keep moving to accommodate more students. I have never done a Sun Salutation where I have been able to fully extend my arms without knocking into someone, and when we're doing Fallen Triangle, my neighbor's foot always ends up on my mat. In yoga, you're supposed to think it's OK for other people to invade your space, and if you're bothered by that, it's somehow your issue. But I would like a little space. I'm not opening my heart if your foot is on my mat.

Once, I just lost it. I said loudly, "It is too crowded in here, and I can't believe I'm the only one who feels that way!" People were looking at me. I got up, went out to the front desk, and said, "The class is packed." They told me, "It's not even full." My reaction was, "*That's* not full?"

Don't get me wrong—I have nothing but respect and admiration for people who do yoga and love it. Yoga bodies are beautiful. I'm even a little jealous of those who excel at it. Me, I find my Zen in other ways.

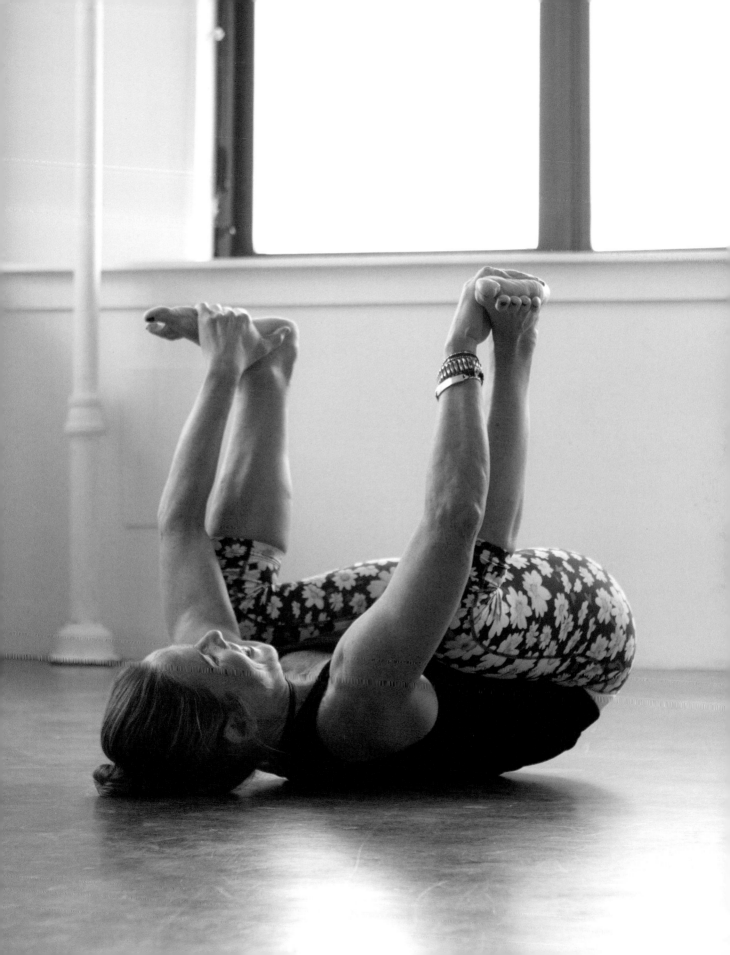

Anna

...

For nearly four years I have been living off my savings and hoping and praying that my yoga-clothing company will take off. I dream the business. I breathe it. I live it. I'm involved with every single aspect, including design, brand-building, sales and marketing, and financial operations.

In my previous job, I was the assistant treasurer at a $28 billion hedge fund, had an incredible amount of resources at my disposal, and was surrounded by extremely talented and smart people. Time was money, and I had to make decisions quickly. I couldn't show weakness. In fact, one of my biggest fears about running my own company was that I would trust the wrong people and it would backfire.

But I have come to realize that vulnerability is an amazing tool in business. People don't talk about it much, but it is true.

Early on, my partner and I realized that a supplier I had hired was dishonest. I felt betrayed and ashamed. There were other big stresses weighing heavily on my shoulders, too, and at the height of it all one afternoon I decided to break away from my laptop and take a yoga class.

Toward the end of class, I just broke down. I realized how hard it was for me to be vulnerable. But I also remember feeling the walls that had been crowding in on me beginning to release. I could look at my situation from a different perspective. It was as clear as day that I could handle the problem of our dishonest supplier. I could move forward, using the wisdom I'd gained from making that mistake. And most importantly, I understood that I had to be a lot more compassionate with myself.

The reality is, if you think people are out to deceive you, then you will manifest that energy, and it will come into your life over and over again. To live the life you want and deserve, you have to trust other people. This trusting-and-letting-go thing is a muscle I have to constantly exercise. But it starts with giving myself permission to be vulnerable, and that realization came to me through yoga.

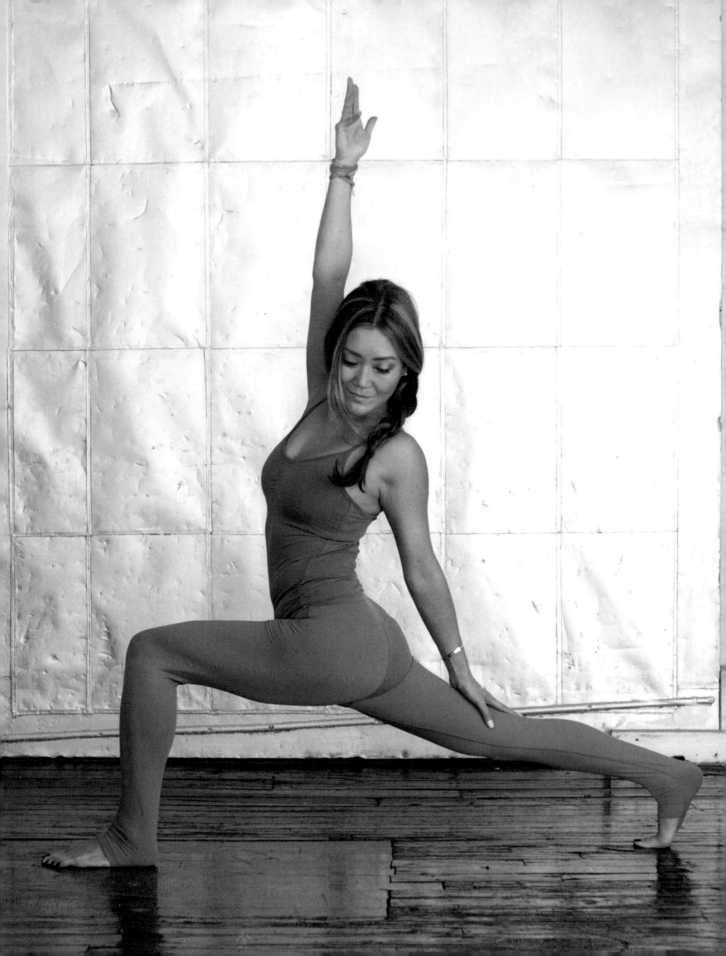

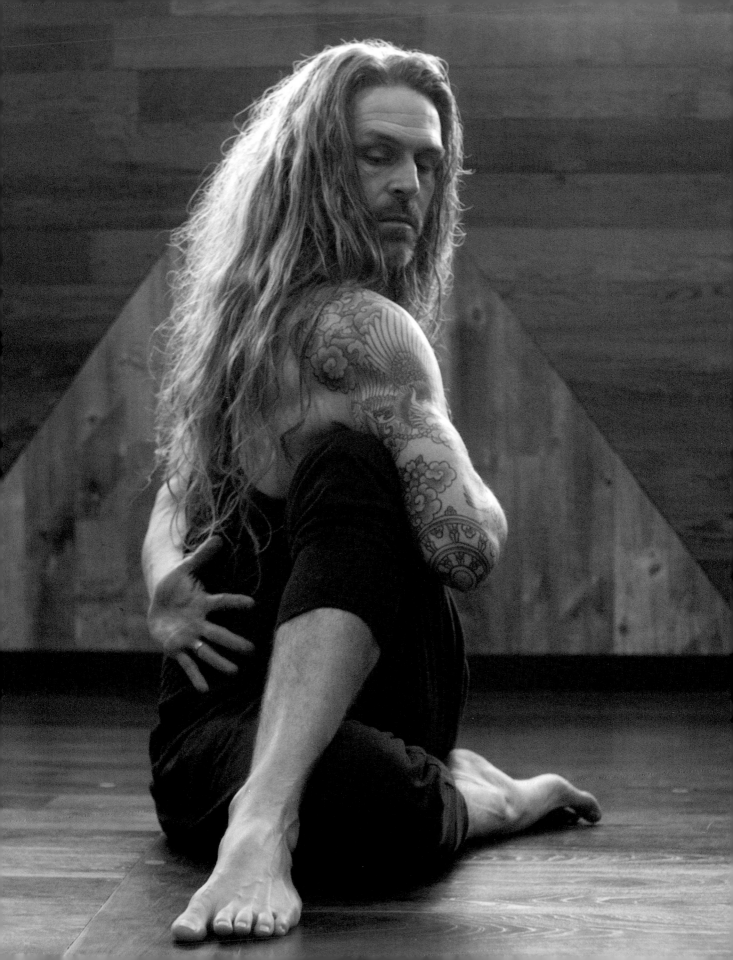

Chad

HALF LORD OF THE FISHES POSE VARIATION

•••

I have a three-year-old son, and this is not a myth: the Terrible Twos and the Absolutely Horrible Threes are phases that really do exist. And I think everything I have been doing in my life up until this point has been to provide me the tools for dealing with a toddler. The last thirty years was the *practice* of yoga; the last three years has been the *application* of yoga.

For most of my life, I was self-absorbed and self-centered, traveling that road of finding out who I was. But my greatest battles and challenges from the past pale in comparison to the challenge of getting my son dressed and out the door in the morning. It is a daily test of patience and compassion and trying to not react in a knee jerk way. I invite any Buddhist monk who's been studying in a monastery for however many years to take care of a three-year-old for few days.

My son just doesn't want to do what Daddy wants him to do: "No, you cannot wear just your underwear to school today. You really can't. And Daddy has to teach a yoga class in forty-five minutes, and we really need to get this show on the road." My son knows all of this and doesn't care. Sometimes I lose my patience and get frustrated. I have to step back, breathe, try not to react, and calmly try to put this kid's socks on.

Change—to me this is what yoga is all about anyway. Yoga is not living in some idealized state. It's about rolling with the punches and hopefully applying whatever techniques we've picked up along the way. Let's be very clear that what you do on the mat for ninety minutes is just one very small part of it. If you walk around the rest of the day disregarding others, you're not doing yoga. You're just doing gymnastics.

Catie

CAT-COW POSE

...

When I was in sixth grade, the cool girl in school took me under her wing. She wore expensive clothes and lots of makeup and used a tanning bed—and this was in middle school! I was the smart, awkward girl who got straight A's and won awards. As you might guess, it turned into the typical mean-girl experience. One night after I'd been hanging out at her house, her mom was driving me home and asked me why I didn't have abs. There are probably other moments that shaped my body image, but I will never forget sitting in the backseat of this van and coming home crying to my mom about why I didn't have abs. I asked for weights for Christmas and started going to the library to rent workout videos.

From that time on, exercise has been about sculpting my body into something better. I still have this weird relationship with my body where after a workout I'll go to the mirror, lift up my shirt, look at my stomach and think, "Is this taking up less space now?"

When I was twenty, I did one of those home-workout boot camp programs: six videos a week for ninety days. It was miserable. I just dreaded every workout. The program has strength training days, cardio days, and a weekly yoga day, and the yoga was the only part of this grueling thing I put myself through that I actually looked forward to. It was the only workout where I wasn't thinking about when it would be over and what I would look like.

Now I'm out of college. I just started a new job and am stressed out of my mind. By the weekend I'm completely exhausted. In the past couple of months I have not exercised, like, at all. But once in a while I'll whip out that yoga video, and when I do it I feel like I'm taking care of myself. I'm not looking in the mirror. For thirty minutes, I'm just listening to my body.

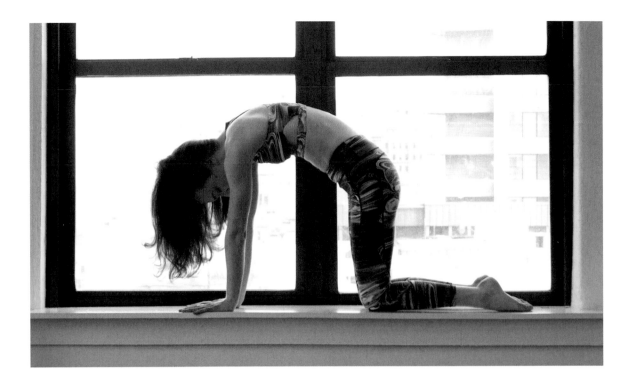

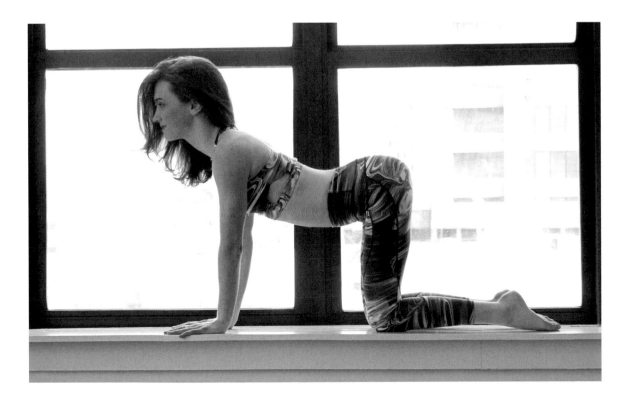

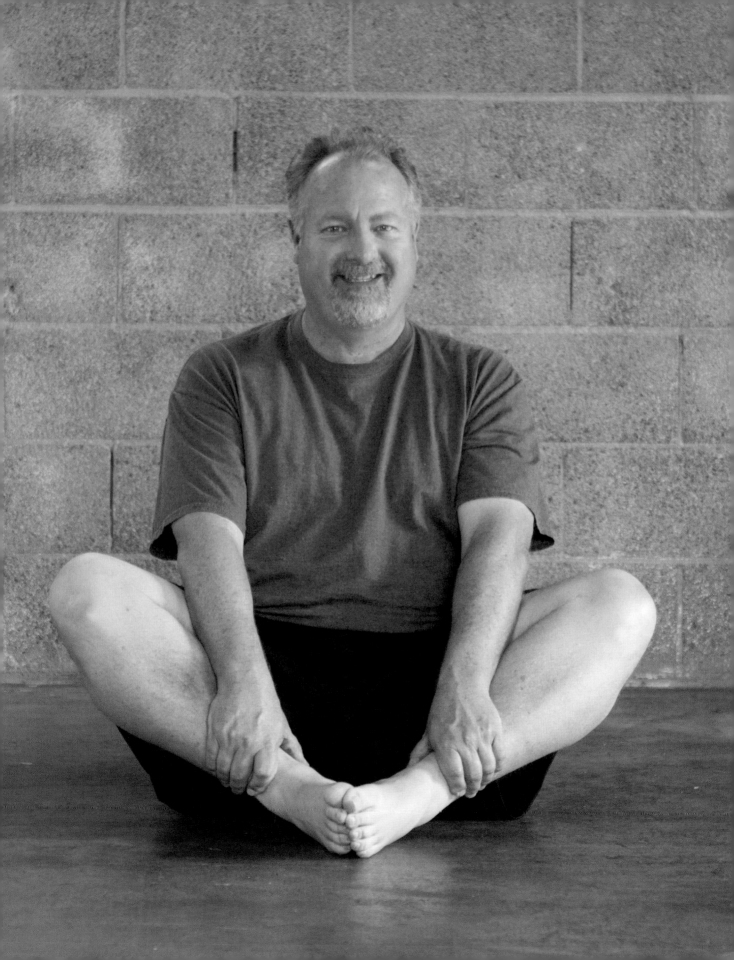

Jeff

BOUND ANGLE POSE

•••

All my life I've had tight muscles. It's a constant battle. My hamstrings and my quads are so tight. My left hip is tight. I have problems with my lower back and my mid-back, up between my shoulder blades. Plus my right rotator cuff has a slight tear in it from playing baseball in a Sunday league.

Lately my fingers and hands have been aching, too. I'm a salesman, so most of the week I'm in my car running appointments. Sometimes I sit in a parking lot and work on my computer. I'll hold the laptop at an awkward angle, and then afterward my hand will be sore. Or I'll reach for my briefcase in the backseat and it tweaks my rotator cuff. All these aches and pains I never had when I was younger . . . it's kind of irritating.

For a while, I kind of got into that Bikram yoga, where they heat the room to 100 degrees or so. The best thing about that was the cool air outside when I left. I know to listen to my body, so I'm not going to go into a yoga pose far enough to hurt myself. I know when enough is enough. But I did notice that with the added warmth it was easier to get into the poses.

Even though I'm not taking classes anymore, yoga has paid off for me. If you put me at a party with a bunch of friends of mine, I'm probably going to be the most flexible person in the room. These days I get up in the morning at least three or four times a week and do my own routine. I'm always looking for a better way to stretch my hip out, and I do exercises for my shoulders.

I'm just in search of a silver bullet that will cure all of my ailments. Do you have one?

Dana

PEACE AND LOVE POSE

...

When I was twenty-five, I opened a restaurant, Trixie's, in Hell's Kitchen, right off of Times Square in New York. It became a huge hit. Madonna, Sandra Bernhard, John Goodman, Cindy Crawford, and even "Trixie" from *The Honeymooners*—they all came. The lines were so long out the door that we had a bouncer. It was a scene, and I was the hostess of the moment and absolutely a party girl.

I had all this success at a young age; I was happy, but my happiness was conditional, and I realized that to last, it had to come from a deeper place. At the height of my partying I turned a cosmic corner and started to investigate more deeply, "Who am I? Why am I here?"—the kinds of questions that make you pick up things like *The Tibetan Book of Living and Dying.* I longed to create a more meaningful life.

I'm grateful now for all of my experimentation, because I wouldn't have found yoga without it.

Now I own my own yoga studio and get to party in a new way.

My style of yoga is vibrant, it's colorful, it's energetic, it's soulful. I weave my passion for philosophy, poetry, and the sacred into every class. The studio has a disco ball and we play a lot of great music to create a positive, uplifting experience for everyone.

I love music: big beats, deep grooves, house, jazz, R&B, everything. I love hearing Aretha wail, and I can't live without Nina Simone. My yoga playlist can include Janis Joplin, Annie Lennox, Fleetwood Mac, a Nusrat Fateh Ali Khan remix, and Mozart, and I might quote a poet like Hafez or Mary Oliver.

I definitely have a lot of enthusiasm for life and love to share it. I live for the energy I feel in a community. I love the coming together. If I could, I would give my classes for free so we could all hang out.

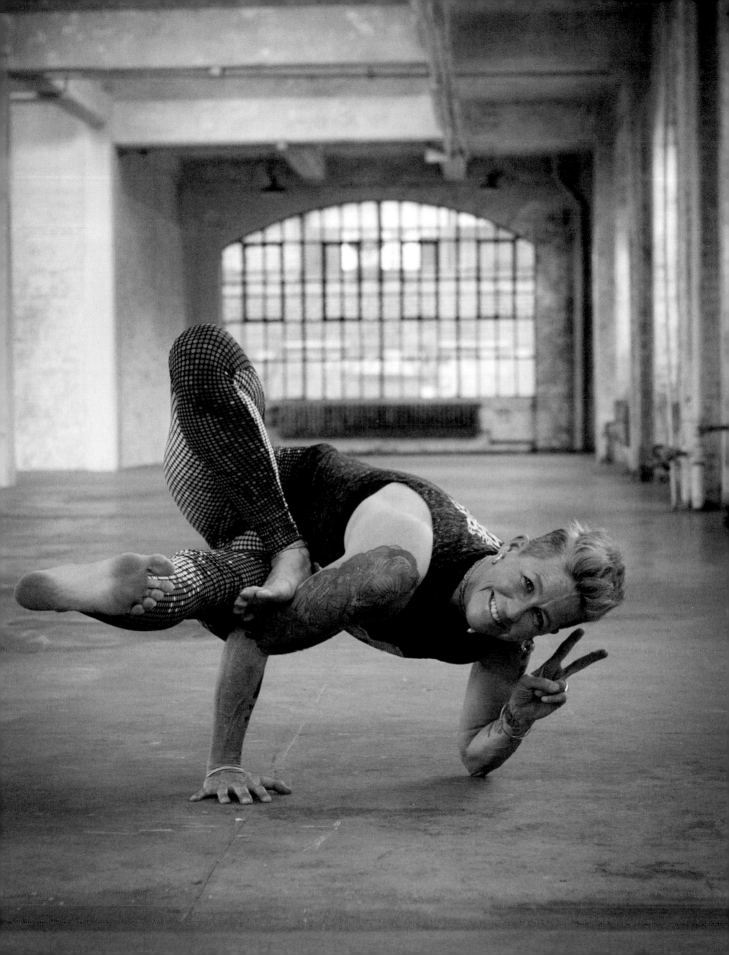

Robyn

GATE POSE

...

Often, as I practice, I repeat a mantra to myself. It might be a reminder to be more patient and less reactive; other times it's about being grateful and feeling love. The mantra can be as simple as mentally telling myself to breathe in and breathe out. After what happened to me, I am so grateful to be able to breathe.

One Sunday two summers ago, after my husband and I had come home from visiting our boys at camp, I noticed my back was bothering me. Every time I took a deep breath, it hurt. I thought maybe I had injured a rib or pulled a muscle. By Sunday night, I couldn't get a full breath in and was in excruciating pain. I went to the emergency room, and as soon as they heard my symptoms, they asked me what kind of birth control I used. It turned out I had multiple blood clots in both of my lungs—a potential side effect of my birth control that is not uncommon, but which I had barely known about. I was in the hospital for six days. It was really frightening. I could have died.

Since then, my whole practice has changed. I used to strive to do every pose the way the teacher did it. Now it's less about "How high is my leg?" or "How flat are my hands on the floor?" It's really about being able to breathe.

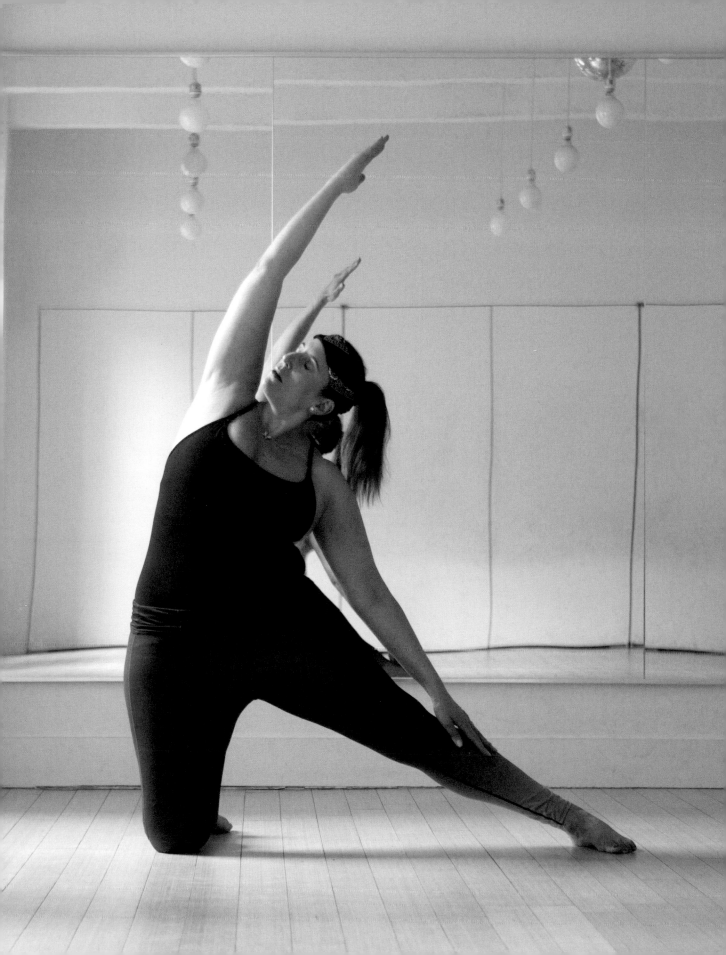

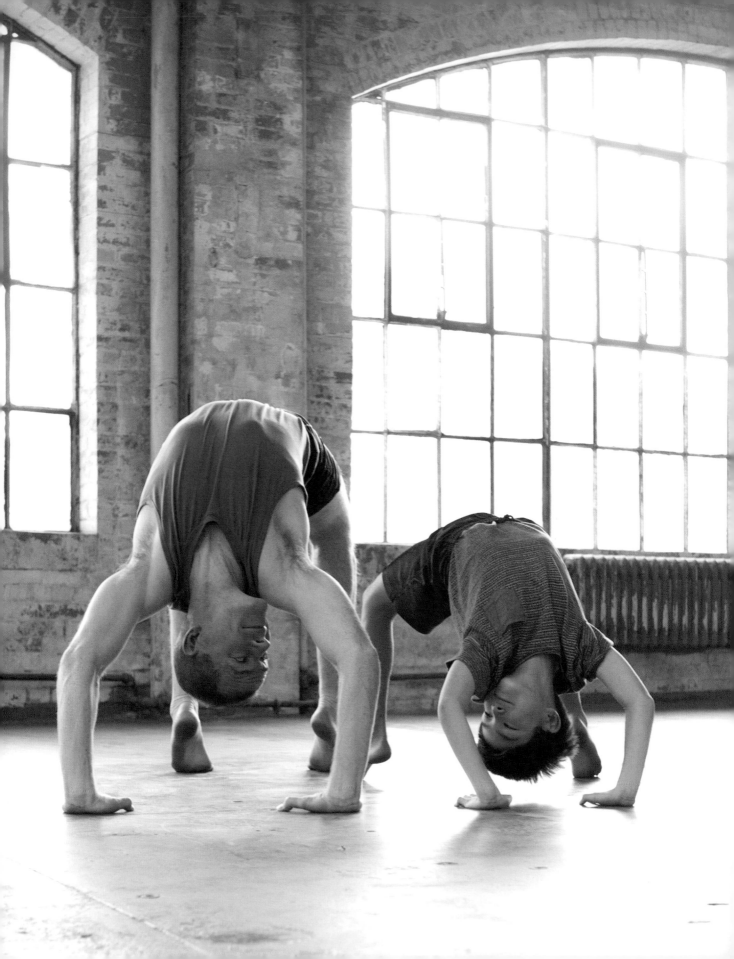

Sean and Tommy

UPWARD BOW POSE

Sean: I have been practicing yoga since just after Tommy was born.

Tommy: I started when I was four.

Sean: A couple of times a month, we'll roll out our mats in the living room. We'll put in a yoga DVD and—I know it's sacrilege—we also might have a game on with the volume down.

We used to do this about once a week, until Tommy started having more activities going on.

Tommy: In the winter I do basketball. In the fall I do flag football, and in the spring I do baseball.

Sean: But yoga is a nice change of pace. Would you say that?

Tommy: Yeah. It's good to relax a little bit. I mean, I'm definitely better at baseball, but if you're good at calming down, you can be pretty good at yoga.

Sean: Sometimes Tommy will correct my form or I'll correct his.

Tommy: It's funny because we both kind of can't do Warrior I. I can't do it my left side, and you can't do it on your right side.

Sean: And lot of the time we're making jokes. The instructor on the DVD says some wacky things: "Soften your belly. Soften your eyes."

He also repeats a lot of sequences, so we'll be like, "Aaaand I believe we've been here before."

Tommy: When we do Upward Bow, he makes you hold it, and then you go back down, and he'll say, "Take five breaths," but you only have time to take two breaths and then you have to go back up.

Sean: So we'll say, "What happened to those five breaths?"

We usually do this on Sundays. My wife doesn't join us—she is interested in yoga, but she's like most of America; she doesn't know where to start. Sometimes my daughter joins in, though.

Tommy: My sister will stay through the first part. You do it over and over again. You go through this series of poses three times, and by then, she will be like, "I'm done."

Sean: Maybe she just doesn't want to hang out with two guys.

Melissa

THREE-LIMBED STAFF POSE

...

I am a yoga and meditation teacher, a Reiki healer and an energy worker. I work with people who have physical ailments or major emotional traumas, like divorce or childhood abuse. I always refer my clients to a psychotherapist as well, but even if they're doing traditional therapy, speaking to someone with just words, the body can still hold negative energy. Our cells lock in trauma, and Reiki and energy work can help clear that out.

When I work with someone, they lie down and I do an energy scan of their body. I hover my hands about two inches above them, usually starting at the crown of their head and working down. Technically I'm scanning all of their chakras. I'll get tingles in my hands or a sharp pain; sometimes I'll get a lot of heat radiating off their body, which indicates that there's a significant amount of *ki,* or life-force energy, in that spot. That's a sure sign of where they're holding trauma. Then I use different techniques to help them move that energy out. I might put crystals on their bodies or flick my hands up and away. As the session progresses, their breath changes and slows, their muscles relax, and they become quiet.

These practices are about opening people's minds to help them know themselves on a deeper level, instead of just going through this life living on the surface. I think about it as snorkeling versus scuba diving. You can snorkel, and the reef looks really good from the top. Or you can put on your scuba gear and dive down, and it might be scary as hell, but you're in the reef and you're with the fish, and it's another whole element. Even in yoga, when you tap into being on your mat, you transition from snorkeling to scuba diving.

I get that some people are skeptical about what I do; I have had clients who come because a friend has referred them, but they're still doubtful. If you create too much of a mental barrier, though, you may not consciously feel the benefits of energy work. Besides, releasing judgment and being open-minded benefit you in so many areas of life. I'm all for people saying, "This is different; I'm not familiar with it, but I'm willing to try it."

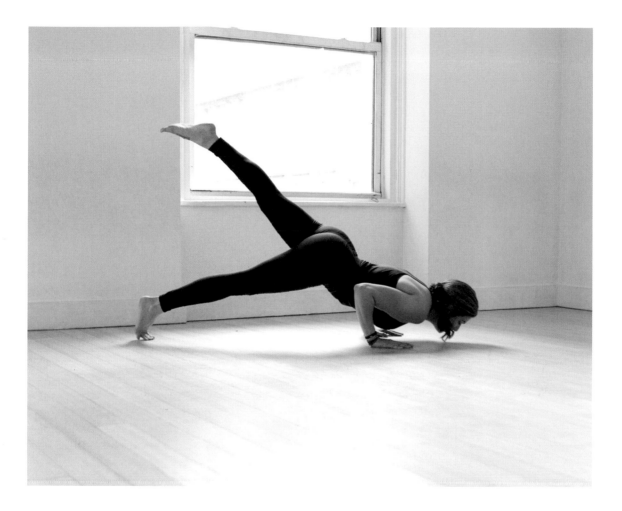

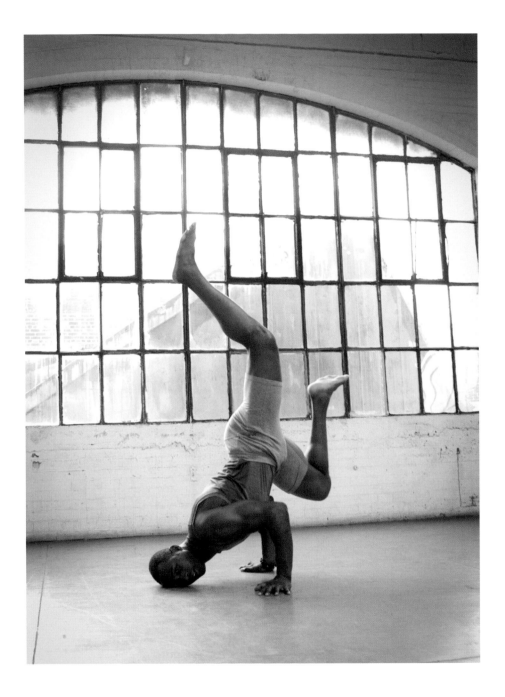

Tony

CHIN BALANCE VARIATION

• • •

There are so many times in a football game when you have to recapture yourself and recommit to yourself. It could be during a long play, when you come back to the huddle winded and have to keep on going. Yoga helped me during those times. When I got fatigued during a game, I'd tell myself, "Breathe. Calm down."

With my current job, yoga helps me be more effective so I don't burn myself out.

I'm retired from the NFL, and now I'm a coordinator for the NFL's Legends Community. We assist players who are retiring, helping them with continuing education, financial matters, medical benefits, job placement, and counseling. For a lot of them the change is emotionally difficult. They go from being someone everybody recognizes to feeling like they're sort of past-tense. I check up on them regularly, and if someone is going through tough times, I can recommend resources to help him.

I try to be there for my friends and family, too. My friends know if they come talk to me, there's no judgment. I hear about finances, marital problems, and work stress. I'm also involved in a lot of charity work, including raising awareness of violence against children.

I guess my interest in helping people goes back to my childhood. My dad was in the military; I was born in Germany, and my parents always opened our home to soldiers there without family. My football career got me into a position where I could give back, and it just snowballed. If I can make a difference, like meeting a kid in the hospital, I will show up. My dad always says, "There are twenty-four hours in a day. What are you going to do with them?"

Yoga is a way to put all of this in perspective. No matter what kind of problems or situations I am dealing with, when I practice, I leave everything on the mat. I walk out of class free from it all and can start all over again.

Caroline

...

When I do yoga, I find peace and freedom and this real, tangible connection to God. I feel how much He loves me, and how proud He is of me.

A lot of Christians are hesitant to go to a yoga class because it feels foreign to them. I am trained in a style called Holy Yoga that fuses the Christian faith with yoga. We don't use Sanskrit names for poses. We wouldn't say *Om,* and we probably wouldn't say *namaste,* not because we think those words are bad, but because our students might be bothered by them. The aim is to remove as many obstacles as possible to appeal to people who wouldn't otherwise walk into a regular class. I know teachers who have tried to start Holy Yoga programs in their churches and were hit with resistance. Still, a lot of times I think Christians are just looking for another Christian to give them permission to do yoga.

When I teach my classes, I always start with a prayer. I'll share a quote from a Christian thinker or author and read scripture that fits with the theme of the class. If the theme is love triumphing over fear, I might read from 2 Timothy: "For God has not given us a spirit of fear, but of power and of love and of a sound mind."

Moving past fear and walking in this spirit of love is what draws me to my mat over and over again. My intention when I practice is to worship God, to enjoy His presence, and to give Him room to speak.

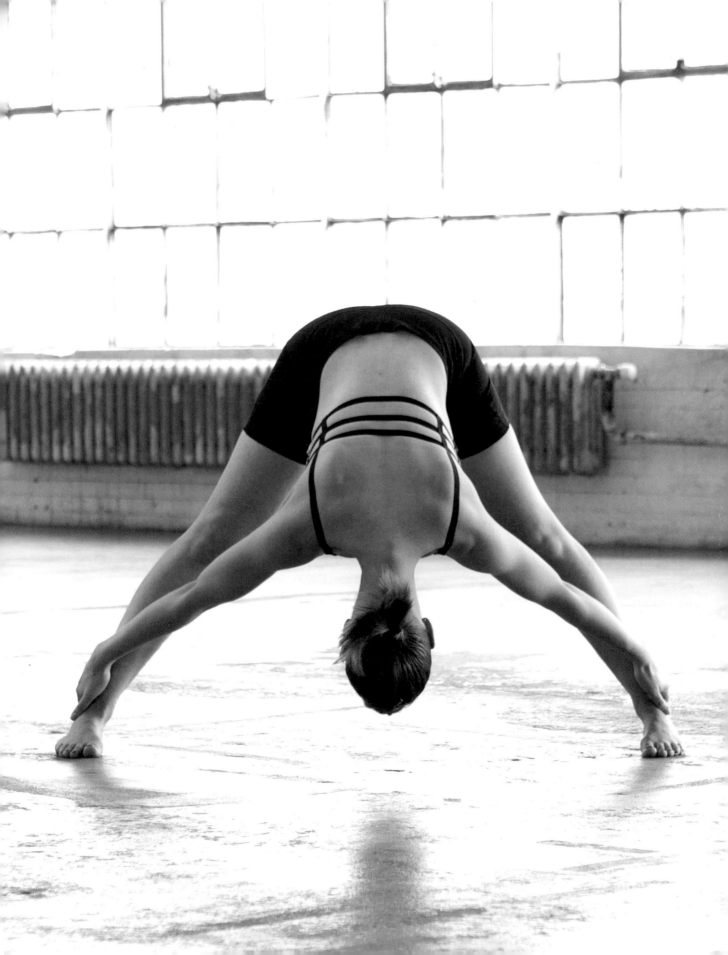

Tanya

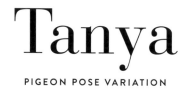

PIGEON POSE VARIATION

•••

I was in a morning yoga class when I felt this overwhelming sensation—like a voice, a push—that said, "Get up and go to the hospital." When I arrived, my dad was Code Blue.

He was seventy and had heart failure and dementia and hadn't been doing well. For two or three years, his health had gotten progressively worse. I was living overseas and had just arrived in Los Angeles to see him the night before. I'd driven straight from the airport to the hospital, where he'd told me, "I was waiting for you." He had been a bit delirious and was saying some things that were quite funny. He hated the hospital and was just like, "Get me out of here!"

We were very, very close. Until then I had never lost someone where it felt like I'd lost a limb. When I realized my father was dying, I was kind of like, "How come life has prepared me for everything else but this? How come the one guarantee in life is death, and no one talks about it?" If you were to make a scale of pain, death is the deepest depth of hurt, and no one talks about how to sit in grief, or how to move on.

Not long after I jolted up from my yoga mat and returned to the hospital, they stopped trying to resuscitate him. When they took the tubes out, I got into bed with him to help take him through to the other side. He was pronounced dead about two minutes later. To watch the spirit leaving the body makes you realize the body is just a unit you're walking around in. I think even when a person dies, their spirit is still with you and around you.

I did get my dad out of the hospital. I got him to a way better place.

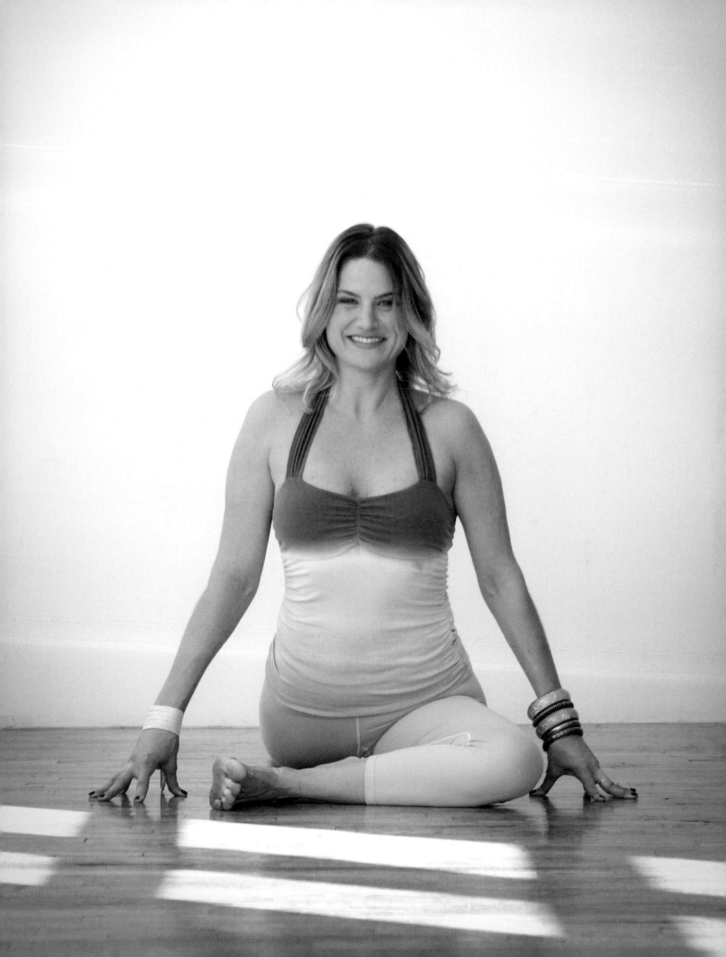

Kay Kay

CRESCENT LUNGE

• • •

I get pissy sometimes, just like everybody else does, when I'm dealing with everyday life and other human beings are pushing my limits. Yoga teaches me to notice when the mind goes there and to bring it back to something positive.

I travel a lot, and things are bound to go wrong when you travel. When I'm delayed at an airport, if there's no yoga room, I'll often find a spot in a corner to practice. I remember being at an airport in Alaska one time and thinking, "I need to do a headstand right now." Another time I was on a flight from Hong Kong, which is already the most awful flight because it's almost twenty hours. On this particular trip there was a baby next to me. The baby was not having a good flight, which meant that no one was having a good flight. I was thinking, "What kind of karma am I being paid back for that I got this seat?"

But I try to remind myself to be compassionate, and whenever I do that, it shifts me. I thought, "That poor baby is uncomfortable," and that made me a little less uncomfortable.

In yoga, when you're in a challenging pose, you've got to surrender to it. If you get yourself worked up, it doesn't help. So you breathe and redirect your energy.

The intention behind yoga is that we're trying to connect with our highest self, the part of ourselves that isn't our ego.

This is what the yoga teaches you: You're strapped into this airplane seat, you're not going anywhere for twenty hours, and this is your reality. There's nothing you can do but find some calm and just deal with it. I'm really lucky to know to take a deep breath and remind myself that we're all doing the best we can.

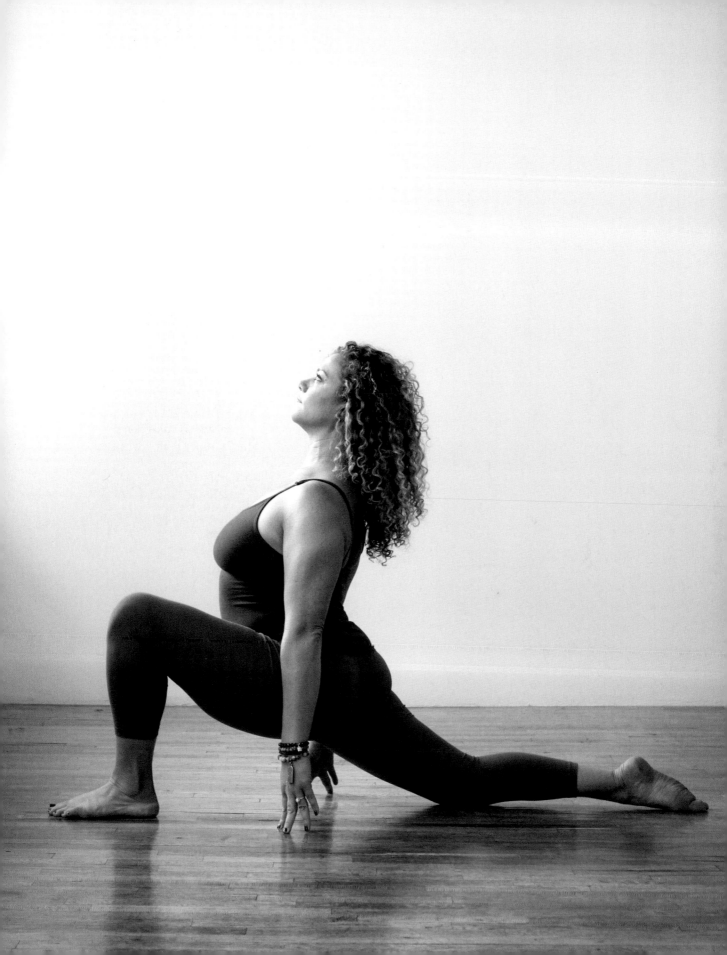

Luke

UPWARD PLANK POSE

...

I had a very long and successful career and retired a year ago, when the biotech company I'd been with for seven years was purchased by a larger company. Until then I was all in at work. I was up at dawn answering emails and in the office by seven-thirty. It would basically be non-stop working until six or seven at night. I'd drive home, have a quick dinner with my wife, and then sit down and do more work until as late as midnight. I would get up the next morning and do it all over again.

There were times when I'd be tired, and, as with any job, there were periods that sucked, but I really enjoyed my work. My company launched two drugs that treat extremely rare diseases, and there are probably ten thousand people in the world today who are either still living or whose lives have improved because of what we did. I was working like a madman, but it was a labor of love.

Now I want to think about how to spend the next phase of my life. I started working four days

after college graduation and never stopped. Now that I finally have the time, I go to the gym every day and to yoga once or twice a week.

All I knew about yoga when I started taking classes was how to spell it. The group setting was intimidating at first; I was definitely out of my comfort zone. Even now, I position myself in a discreet corner of the room because I'm so insecure. My body's bigger, I'm fifty-seven, and half the time I'm the only guy in the class. I also don't know a lot of the names of the moves.

In my executive role, I was always thinking about the entire organization and was very aware that my every action would have an effect on the company and the people in it. In yoga, all I'm thinking about is me—the pose I'm doing, and whatever is going through my mind—stuff that in my former day-to-day routine I didn't have time to think about. And, frankly, I know nobody is looking at me. It's the antithesis of what I have been doing for the last thirty years, and it's great

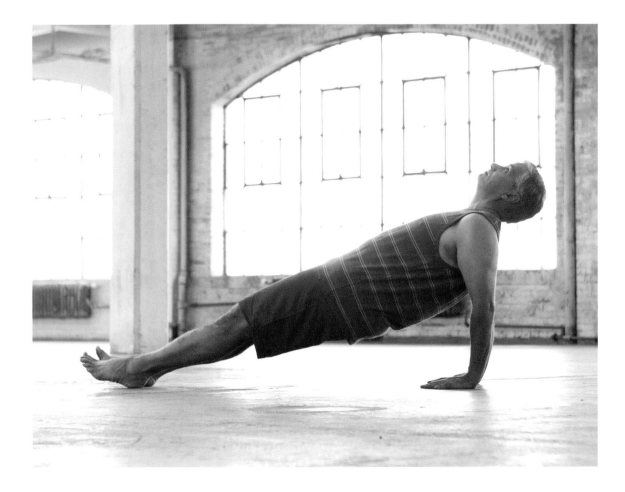

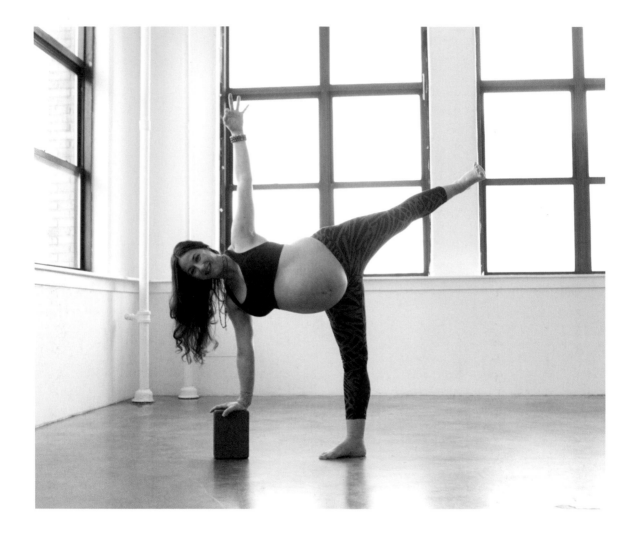

Sheri

HALF MOON POSE

...

As my pregnancy has progressed, I have found that I'm still capable of doing so many poses. I have flexibility, I have strength, I can go upside-down, and my hips are really open. The most interesting part of the experience has been that even though I *can* do these things, I have made the choice to rein it in. I'll think, "OK, I don't need to indulge my ego and do a handstand scorpion in this class of sixty people when I'm forty-one and pregnant." I could be hardcore if I chose to, but instead I want to soften.

Lately I've been into *metta* meditation. *Metta* is a word that means loving-kindness.

When you do this meditation, you sit quietly and radiate those feelings out to the world. You start with yourself: "May I be happy and free; may my baby be happy and healthy and free." Then I add my husband and people who are close to me: "May they be happy and free." Then I include the city, and then maybe people who are challenging to me: "May they be happy and free and safe from harm." You keep going and expanding that wish to everyone, to all beings. For the most part that's been my yoga practice lately.

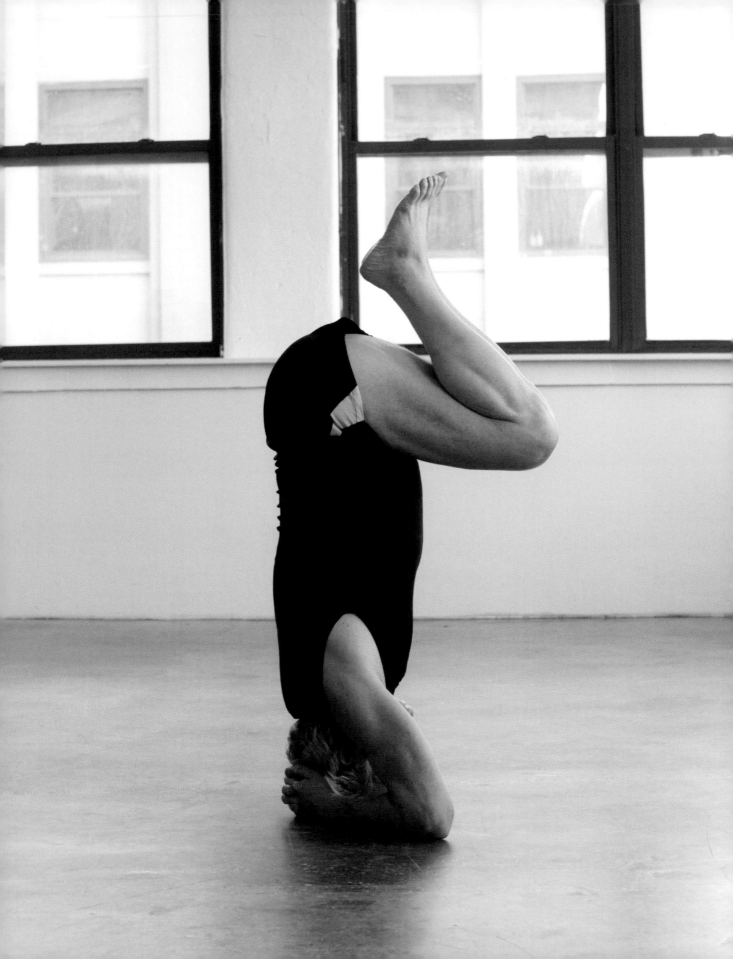

Jim

...

Nearly all sighted people are captives to their sight. They think what they see is reality, but they use their sight to evaluate and judge the world based on some arbitrary standard. As a blind person, it is my experience that how things feel, not how things look, matters most.

What if a pose does not look "amazing," based on the viewer's criteria? Would that diminish the experience of the yogi doing the pose?

If the pose looks horrible, should the yogi consider his or her experience less than adequate?

For people who possess the gift of sight: Just remember that it is often your attachment to what you consider beautiful that defines your experience. The blind yogi must work to develop an evenness of mind that transcends the polarities of right/wrong, beautiful/ugly, adequate/deficient.

Sighted people see my disability and then graft onto it their own opinions of blindness. Nearly all of the time, those judgments are not positive. There is no changing them, no matter how those of us with disabilities may try.

It is we who must dive deeper into ourselves with the faith that we might one day revel in our own world of beauty, free of external evaluations, whether positive or negative.

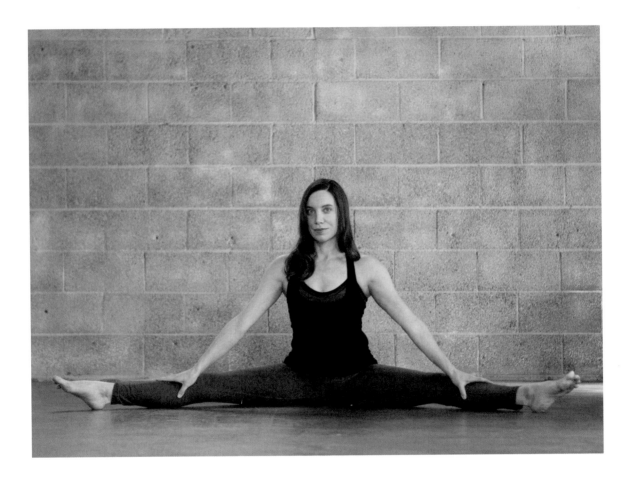

Summer

WIDE-ANGLE SEATED POSE

•••

People contact me all the time and say, "If you need more material for your show, let me know and I'll give you stories." One woman recently told me about an experience she had on a yoga retreat I led years ago: she woke up in her room and one of her suitemates—a fellow yogi—was going through her stuff. These real-life antics are why the series is so relatable: even in the yoga world, people are people, and people are flawed.

Namaste, Bitches is a six-episode web series about an up-and-coming yoga teacher who moves from New York City to Los Angeles to break into the Hollywood yoga scene. She is given a tryout at a mom-and-pop studio, where the other teachers really don't want her to succeed because it will take away from their own followings. She tries to win students over any way she can, to her own detriment. The characters stab each other in the back, smoke, and sleep with their students. They're mean and unforgiving. It's a dark comedy about the underbelly of the yoga world.

When I wrote the series, I heightened some of the elements for comedic effect, but I also drew from very, very, very specific moments in my own career as a yoga teacher. The yoga scene can be brutally competitive. There's really no way to get around that, especially when you create a business out of it.

The first time we did a reading of the script, one of the actors was horrified: she couldn't imagine her yoga teacher would do any of these things. But three of the other stars, who are also yoga teachers in Los Angeles, were not shocked at all. It's not easy to make a living teaching yoga.

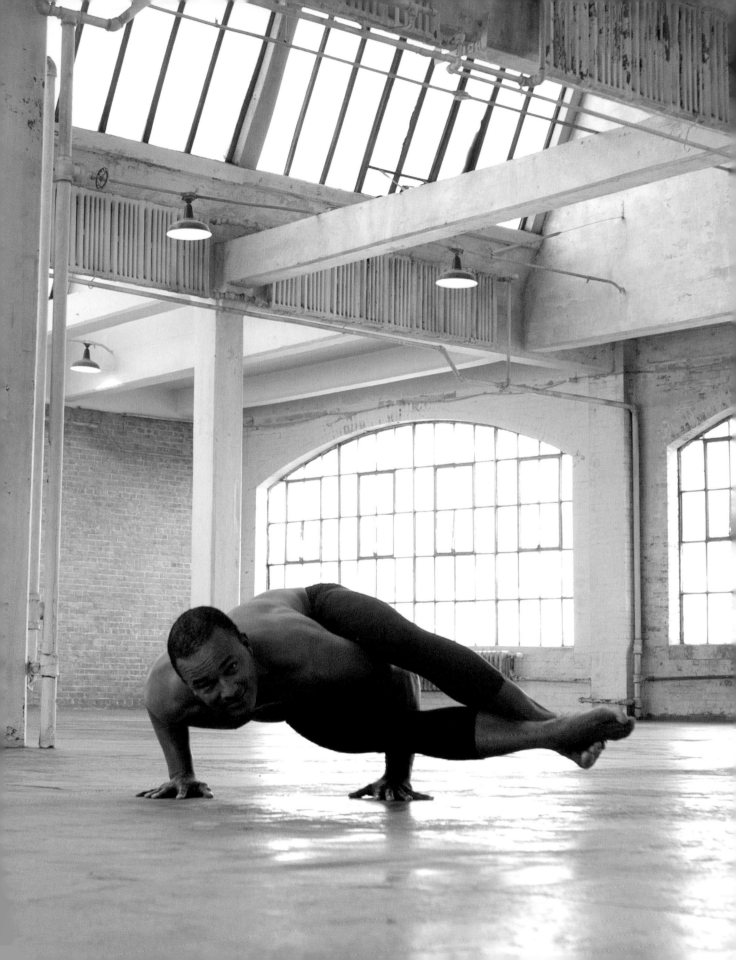

Jay

EIGHT-ANGLE POSE

· · ·

I try to get to the yoga studio twice a day, before and after work, but all of that can get blown out of the window, because there's no typical day in transplant surgery. Transplants can come in at any time. You have to be ready at a moment's notice.

Tomorrow morning, I'm going to Maryland to procure a liver for one of my patients in the Bronx. I'll wake up around five and get to my hospital about six. An ambulance there will take me and a few other doctors and residents to Teterboro Airport in New Jersey. These surgeries have time constraints that don't always work with commercial airline schedules, so we'll use a private plane. When we land, another ambulance will be there to take us to the hospital in Maryland where there will be a donor waiting.

An organ donor is a person who has just died—who has no more blood flow to the brain, but whose body is being kept alive on a breathing machine. We keep their identities anonymous, but this one is a young person who died

from asthma, basically. The patient's family has graciously allowed their loved one to be a donor, which is an unbelievable act of kindness for society and the world.

There might be a few different medical teams in Maryland tomorrow. I specialize in liver, kidney, and pancreas transplants, but there might also be a heart team there, and a lung team, and others. Sometimes when we land at an airport we'll see three or four other planes there from all over the country. You all sort of bond over this shared experience.

In the operating room, it's always solemn before we begin to remove the organs. We honor the donor with a moment of silence. Sometimes a nurse will read a written statement from the family; the family will write about how lucky they are to have lived with their loved one, and how they are passing on this gift to other people. It's heart wrenching and connects everyone in the room. At that moment you're not a surgeon; you're a

CONTINUED NEXT PAGE

human being in this beautiful circle of life.

Surgery feels like an athletic event sometimes. I hydrate a lot and wear compression socks, and I'll even do some yoga on the plane to make sure my posture's OK. Still, your muscles get tired, your back hurts, and your neck hurts. It can be tough to press through, and sometimes it feels like the world is working against you. Transplant surgery is a very humbling practice. Things can happen with patients' immune systems or infections that are out of your control. But there are a lot of people helping you along the way. And maybe you get some help from the universe.

Tomorrow, I'll perform the surgery to remove the liver and bring the liver with me, and we will all get back into an ambulance. It will be lights-and-sirens to the airport: The liver won't last more than ten hours, so we will be in an emergency situation. We'll be given priority and take off immediately. Everyone is in on the mission—the pilots, too. These guys fly in and out of some very bad weather, and planes have gone down with medical teams in them. I always tip my hat to the pilots.

We will land back in New Jersey, take another ambulance to my hospital where the recipient will already be in the operating room, and start the transplant. Most of our liver patients have had cancer or have hepatitis or autoimmune disease, and you're literally changing their lives. These people become like family to us. It's the most beautiful thing when, a year later, you're walking in the hall with coffee in your hand, and a patient stops you to say, "Thank you so much," and you just hug it out.

The biggest thing yoga teaches you is to be present and focused, which helps, obviously, during an operation. But it also reinforces the art of practicing empathy and compassion for yourself and for other people around you. Yoga makes me a better person and a better doctor for sure.

But tomorrow will be a long day. I probably won't make it to yoga.

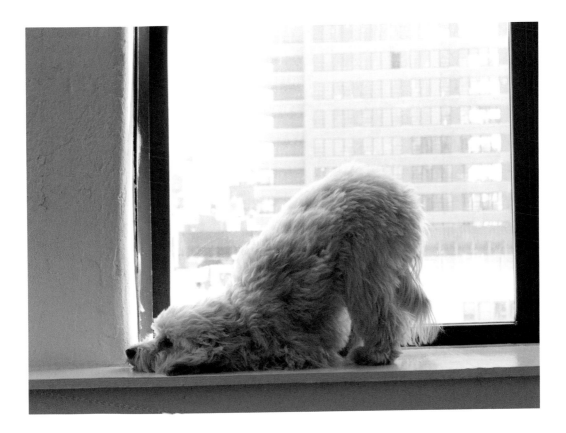

Sunny

DOWNWARD-FACING DOG POSE

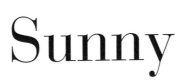

Viji

WARRIOR I POSE

...

Yoga is part of life in India. It's a practical philosophy involving every aspect of a person's being, and it is intended to make life as efficient and enjoyable as possible. Even in school we used to have yoga; as soon as we finished assembly, we would have this exercise regimen.

Today, it's part of my daily routine, like brushing my teeth. I may not look very thin and streamlined, but because of yoga, I can walk fast, I can run, and I can sit for more hours. I am a university professor, and I can stand straight when I give a lecture to my students.

But I don't see yoga as a physical discipline alone. I see it as a spiritual discipline, a selfless service that you are doing for yourself. Any kind of stretching and meditation in the morning goes a long way toward making your day fruitful.

Yoga started as an Eastern practice, and now it has traveled far and wide, and people in the West are taking more interest. Some people call that cultural appropriation, but yoga has far-reaching benefits, so why should there be a divide? Yoga is bigger than that. It cannot be restricted to a certain caste, creed, region, or country. It is meant for mankind, like food, shelter, or clothing. Yoga is universal.

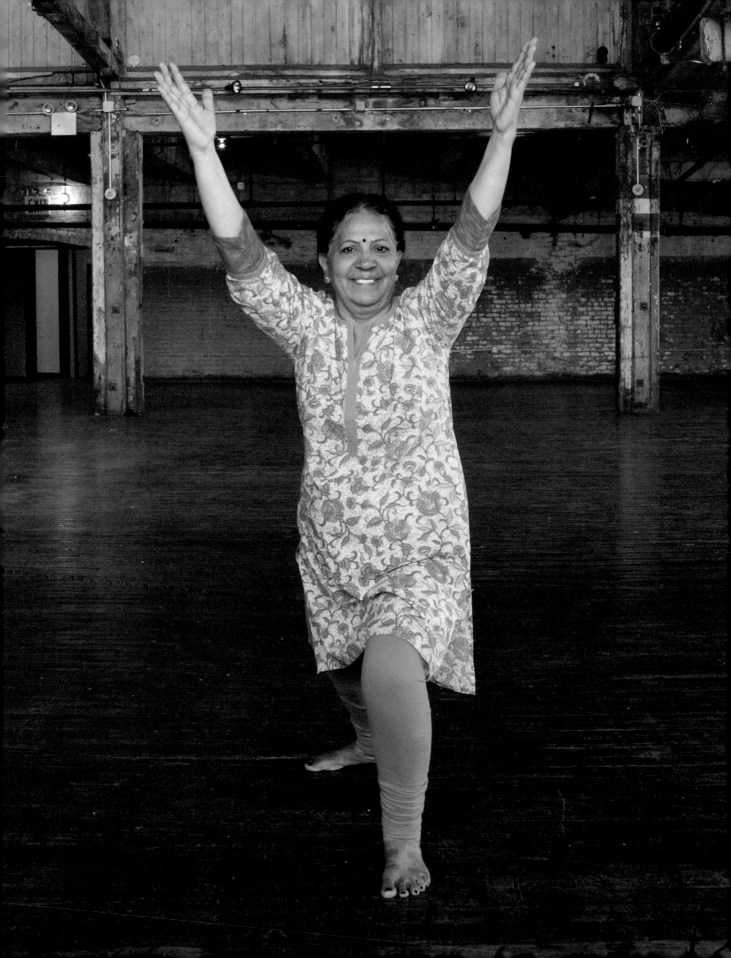

Ryan

FLYING PIGEON POSE

...

Working as an assistant director on TV commercials affords me a good living. I love the process; I love the people. I just don't like the end result. I am helping sell discontentment and the false idea that there is this external thing—be it an air freshener, a cell phone plan, a car—a thing you can pay for that will make you happier. I realized this a couple of years ago and thought, "What am I doing to people? Why am I putting my time and energy and effort into this activity I ultimately don't agree with?"

So I do plan on transitioning out at some point. Doing commercials has provided me with the income and flexible schedule I need to attend yoga teacher trainings. I am currently doing a teaching apprenticeship, which I consider my night school. When I am however old, fifty or fifty-five, and hopefully have been financially responsible enough to have saved some money, I will lead retreats or own a studio.

Right now, my concern is: How can I bring my yoga onto a commercial film set? I'm managing a crew of seventy people; how can I be present for them? And how can I conduct my life in an ethical and conscious way? I was on a job last week and noticed there was less meat served on set, and the craft service girl told me it was because she'd become a vegetarian. I thought about casual conversations she and I have had in the past—I became a vegan as part of my yoga practice—and I don't know, but maybe those conversations influenced her decision in some way. Other times my coworkers come to me and say their lower back is hurting, and ask me for some stretches.

Some people joke about it. If I get stressed on a set, people are like, "What's going on, Yoga Man? Not staying calm?" I'll think, "They're right," and work on settling myself down.

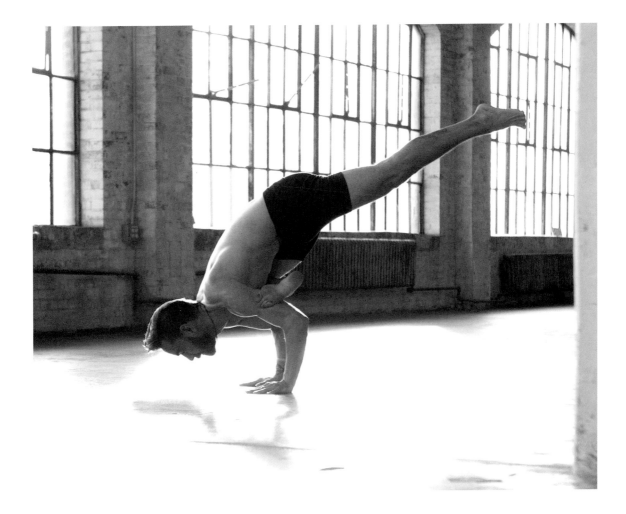

Katie

EXTENDED SIDE ANGLE POSE VARIATION

. . .

After my mom died I wrote a book about her, so I lived with her death as a central character in my personal and professional life for three years. I made an inward promise to her that once the book was done, I would find a way to let go of her death. When the book was published, though, it was: full stop. You're writing it, and then you're doing talks about it, and then it's over. I had a void in my life, but I had to make good on this promise, and I became very depressed.

I had done some yoga before; it was when my mom was sick, actually. I'd wanted to like it then but didn't. I could not stand the quiet. At that time yoga was not an escape for me. It was too emotionally, physically, and spiritually intense.

But after the book came out, I had gained a little weight and felt sedentary. I heard about a hot-yoga studio near my house that played really good music, so I went to a class and stood at the back of the room.

It was hot, it was dark, it was loud, and I loved it. Since then I have never not had a regular practice. There's no style of yoga that I won't try.

My mom did yoga sometimes, but Pilates was mainly her thing. Long before Pilates was in vogue, we had a reformer machine in our house. I thought it was so embarrassing—my mom and her Pilates. My sister and I have pictures of her doing Pilates outside. My mom and stepdad would go to the beach for the summer, and she would schlep the reformer to their little rented condo, put it on the deck and do Pilates out there every day. She would want us to take pictures, and we'd be like, "Ugh, Mom!" It was so annoying. Now, when I make my husband take pictures of me doing yoga, he says, "This is exactly what you used to roll your eyes about." My mom was the original exercise show-off.

In some ways I feel like yoga is time with my mom. I feel like she's with me when I do it, that she's so proud of my fitness and my grace and my commitment to it. We didn't share it together in real life, but I know we are sharing it now. It's amazing how something can connect you to a person who died before you even started practicing it.

126

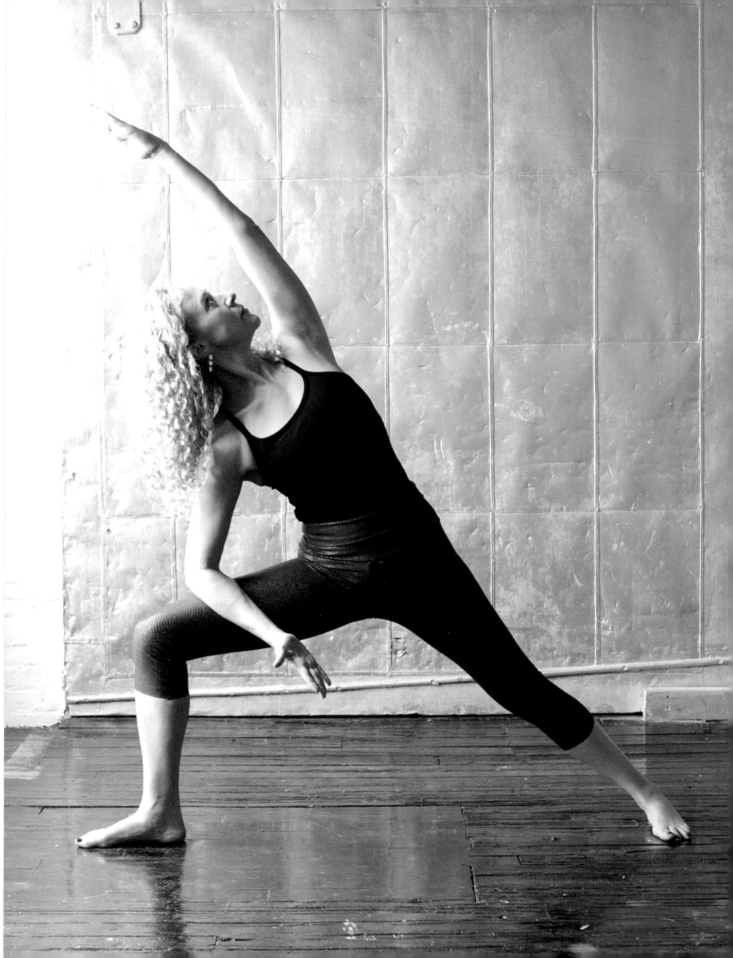

Benjamin

TREE POSE VARIATION

...

A lot of yogis insist that theirs is the One True Path. It's so silly, so tribal. Nothing puts you back in high school quite like reading the comments on a yoga blog. It's a parade of students parroting their teachers parroting their gurus about the unique and superior attributes of this particular style or that one. "Real yogis don't use mirrors." "In yoga there's no ego." "You can't do real yoga if you aren't following the *yamas* and *niyamas*" (a yogic analogue to the Ten Commandments).

All these "don'ts" don't work for me. If you even scratch at yoga history, if you open a single book not written by a self-interested guru, you'll see that there is no single tradition. Yoga is varied and vibrant and really, truly weird. There are militant yogis, mercenary-assassin yogis, and yogis who chained themselves to rocks for years practicing austerity. There are plenty of meat-eaters (to say nothing of urine-drinkers). And so I have no sympathy for people who denigrate other styles. I follow many of the *yamas* and the *niyamas* as a way of life—nonviolence, truthfulness, self-study—but the fact that I don't follow them all doesn't make my practice less "real."

This quest for authenticity reflects where we are right now. We don't have a deep connection to tradition, so the idea of ancient knowledge is tremendously appealing. But a procession of gurus passing down knowledge from one to the next through the centuries, and then that getting delivered to you in your Spandex on your mat on an incense-scented Sunday afternoon—that's a pipe dream. Or a marketing tool.

This is not to say that I think yoga should be an Americanized buffet where each person picks though the history of yoga and cobbles together their own style. Form, discipline, unity within each posture and within an overall practice—these seem like powerful vital concepts to me. I don't want to lose them.

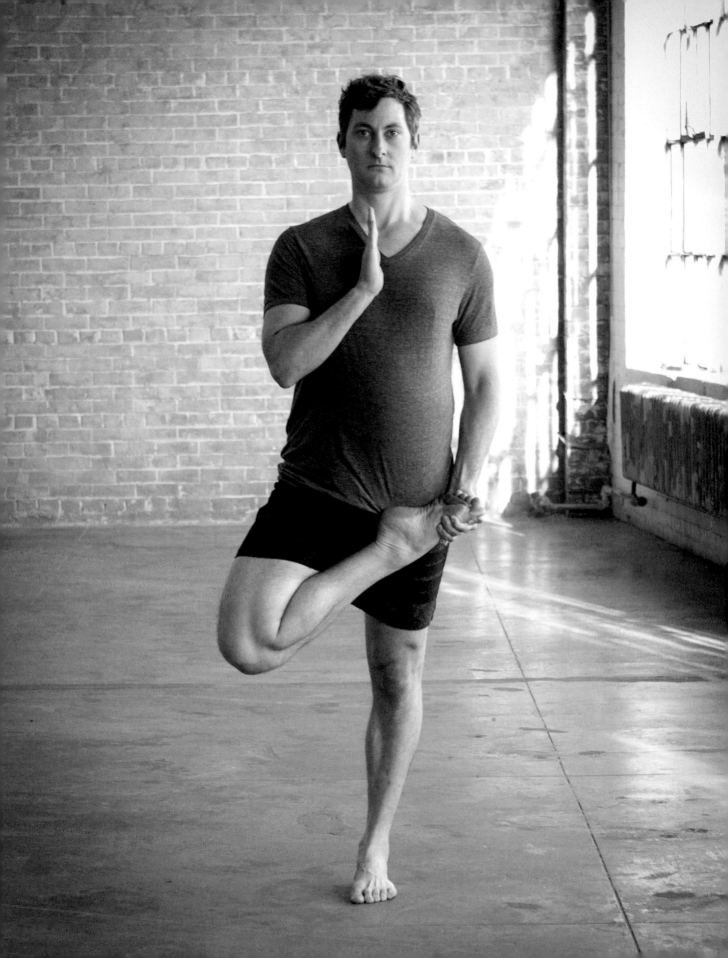

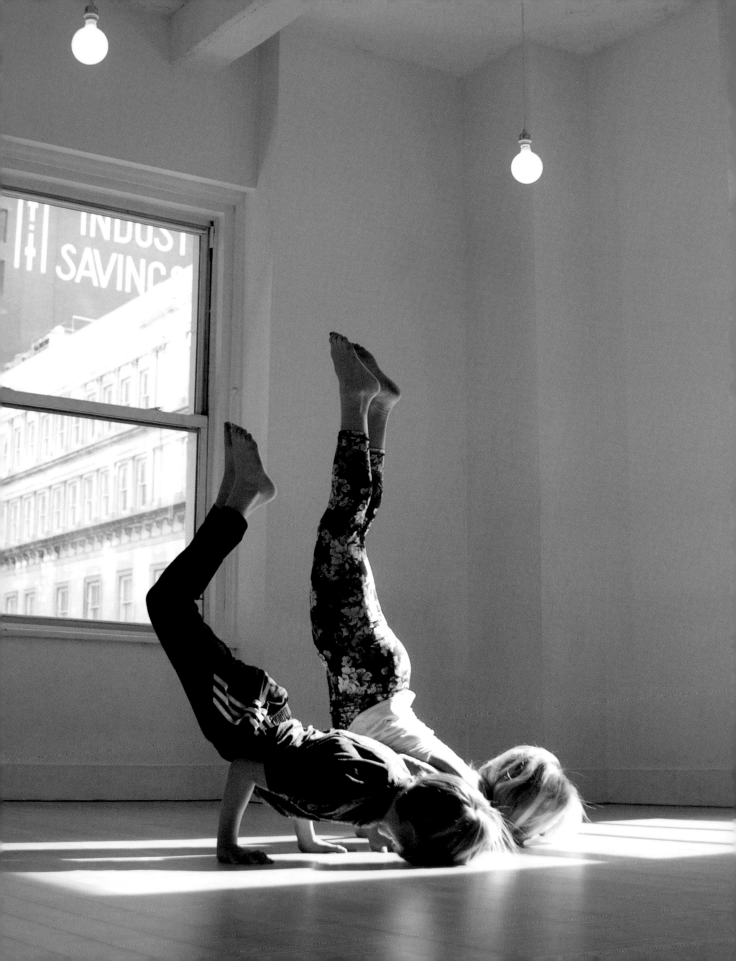

Sam and Jen

CHIN BALANCE

• • •

Jen: My son and I are similar in many ways. We both sometimes have a low threshold for frustration. I'm the type of person who gets impatient on long lines and annoyed at taxi drivers when they go the wrong way. That often comes across in my tone of voice and body language. I get over whatever is bothering me in seconds, but I know it affects the people around me for longer. It's something that I'm trying to work on.

Sam can be the same way, and this particular day didn't start great for us. I thought bringing him with me to this photo shoot would help him shake it off. Sam doesn't do yoga, but he takes break-dancing lessons. I knew he could do a Chin Balance but didn't realize he could hold it

so long. As he got into the pose, his personality came out.

Posing together for this photo just washed away the entire day's frustration. Now it's like a whole new day for both of us.

Sam: I was tired, but I came along with my mom, thinking, "This is going to be interesting for her. It's a new experience."

My mom does yoga all the time, so I know she's really good at it, but I was really surprised when she did this pose with me. When she sees me break dance she always says, like, "Sam, you're so great. I could never do that."

But most mothers can't do poses like this. I didn't know she could do it. It was very cool.

Susan

HALF LORD OF THE FISHES POSE

...

The first time someone suggested I use the ladies' locker room was at my yoga studio. I'd change in the men's room, and the men in there would see me putting on my clothes and a little makeup after class. One day, one of the teachers said, "You know, you can use the ladies' room." I thought he was joking, but he wasn't. I decided to try it.

I went in and then ran out.

I was just so overwhelmed. I hadn't stopped to think that the women would all be without clothing. I saw naked bodies, my heart started pounding, and I was like, "Oh, my god!" One of the locker room attendants was laughing hysterically. She said, "You're so funny; you ran out of there like a little kid!"

In my mind, I am a woman, just as much as any other woman. I have never felt like a man. I have tried to suppress it, but it doesn't go away. The women in the locker room knew me already from yoga class. They knew I am transgender. I practice in a sports bra, tights, and nail polish. But I was so scared to take that next step and use the ladies' locker room.

Two days after I ran out, I decided to try again. This time, the studio manager said, "I'll walk in with you if you want." She and I went in there together, and this time, I kid you not, the women came up to me and said, "Congratulations!" At least six or seven of them gave me hugs. They said, "Welcome. Look; you're one of us now."

Now it's, like, amazing. I come in, and they go, "Hey, Susan." Everyone says hello. I do stay wrapped in a towel so nobody sees any parts, and I notice that once in a while, a lady here or there will move away from me into another area of the locker room. I understand. I wish sometimes I could talk to them, to explain how much I want to be accepted.

But overall, the yoga studio has been one of the most receptive places I have ever been to. It's not a problem for people there. Yogis are very much like, "No big deal. We love you."

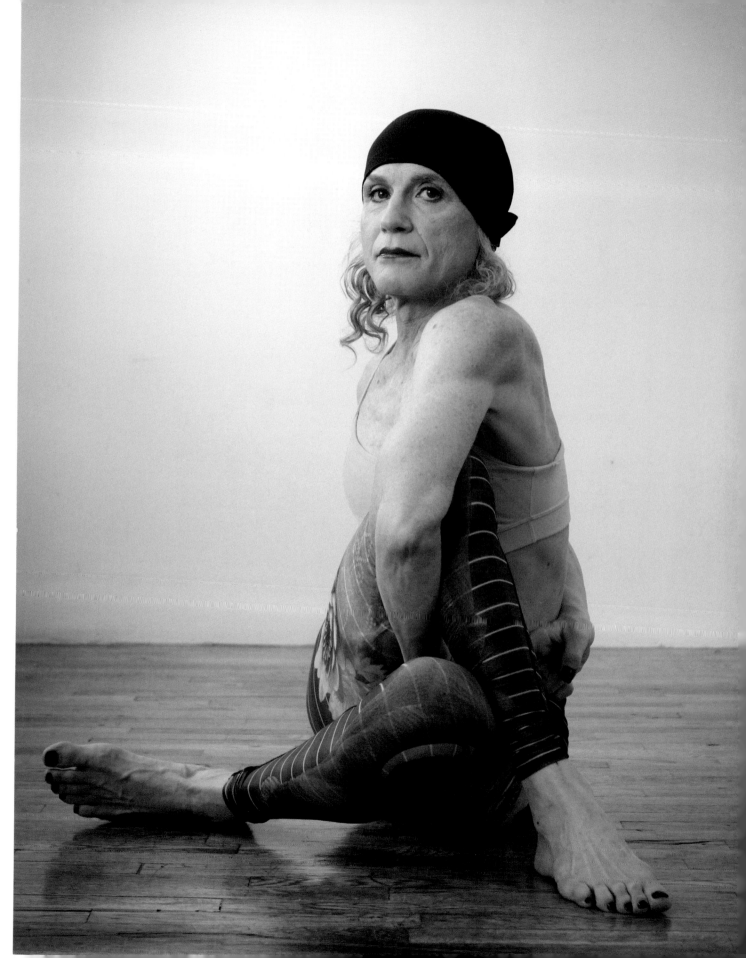

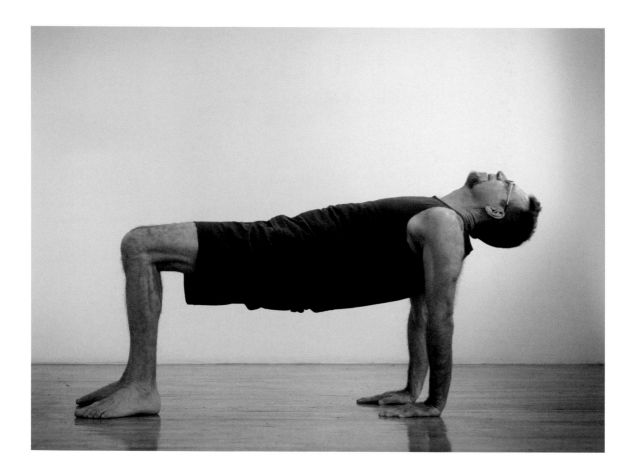

Jeff

UPWARD TABLETOP POSE

...

I originally started doing yoga to help my back and my running. I notice the physical effects more with my back: I'm stronger and more flexible now, and I've firmed up my core.

But I think yoga has also improved my focus. At the end of class we meditate for a little bit, which I think comes into play during the running.

A marathon is a mental game: mind over body. For the first half of the race, I'm enjoying the scenery and the crowds who scream my name for encouragement. (A lot of runners wear shirts with their names on them.) There's lots of music playing in the streets, which pumps me up as well.

By the thirteen-mile mark, it begins to get a bit tough. I have a bad knee, and the pain comes and goes. At this point, I start to break down the race into smaller segments, which eases the daunting task of getting through another thirteen miles.

The training, too, is grueling. Starting four months beforehand I run five to six days a week, including three twenty-mile runs. Sometimes I'm out for three hours or so, but I get a kick out of going long distances. There's a meditative quality to them as well.

I run alone, without music, and concentrate on the surroundings, the scenery, the feel of the air. I focus on my body, think about things that are going on with life, and find solutions to problems.

I run because I really love setting goals. The competition is with myself—to improve my stamina, strength, and time. With life, with work, with family, relationships, what's the point if you're not striving to improve?

There is a goal within the yoga, too. It helps me get where I want to be.

Denise

BOUND HALF MOON POSE

•••

Yesterday during class, I noticed one of the other students staring at me. Afterward, she came up to me. She said she'd only been doing yoga for three weeks and was like, "How do you do all of those things?"

The answer is, by practicing every day, for fifteen years.

Yoga is really time-consuming. You're not going to get it in ten hours, ten thousand hours, or a hundred thousand hours. But when you put effort and thought into it, it's rewarding. I don't have to think about the poses as much as I used to; I just do them. There's something liberating about that.

Not that I can do every pose. I'm thinking it might take me twenty years to be able to press up into a handstand, and there are some things my body will probably never be able to do.

I'm at peace with that. Ten years ago, I wasn't at all.

And after a while, the revelations get really subtle. Recently I was talking to one of my teachers about my Warrior II, because she keeps coming over to me in class and making the same adjustment. I said to her afterward, "I feel like I just don't understand Warrior II," and she explained that I should be using my leg muscles in a slightly different way.

I had never thought of that, and it made total sense. To me those revelations are pretty elusive, but they're why I stick with it.

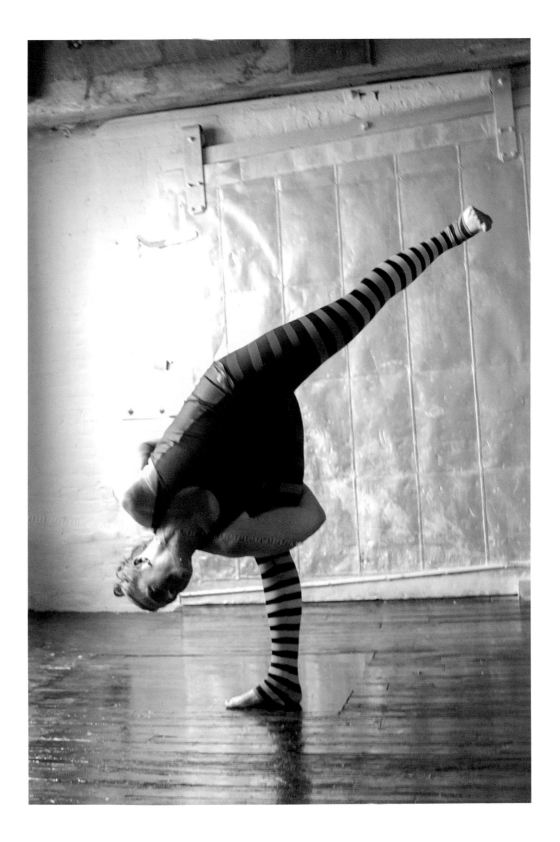

Kiley

FIREFLY POSE

...

I remember in college lying down in the street for peace, being proud of my protests and civil disobedience, and thinking it was very important.

I had hoped to be a professor. As an under-grad, I studied the history of U.S. foreign policy. This was in the early 2000s, at the time of the Iraq War, and I became very interested in how the American people did or didn't understand the United States' involvement in the world. It was really almost an activist heart that brought me to the field of diplomatic history: I wanted to help people know how to ask the right questions.

So I went to graduate school for a PhD. And, you know, it was hard. It wasn't a cheery topic, and it weighed on me. I also found myself wondering if my being a history professor was going to make a difference. I was disheartened by the state of the nation and doubted whether I could do anything about it as an academic.

Meanwhile I had gotten very into yoga. I had begun a daily practice when I was twenty-four.

What initially appealed to me was that it cured me of the insomnia and depression I had been grappling with for over a decade. Later, I loved it for teaching me important life lessons through the movement of my own body. I learned the value of having discipline while still remaining detached from the outcome of my work.

I ended up leaving academia and becoming a yoga teacher. I don't think there's anything wrong with the fact that I was planning on getting a PhD and now use pretty much none of my studies. I don't regret for a single day my advanced education, not because I'm more interesting at somebody's cocktail party, but because it makes me a richer, fuller yoga teacher. I don't think that's lost on my students.

I do feel like I'm making the world more peaceful. I don't lie down in the street anymore. But when fifty people are lying down at the end of a yoga class, that is lying down for peace. It's taking a holy moment. I think that is powerful.

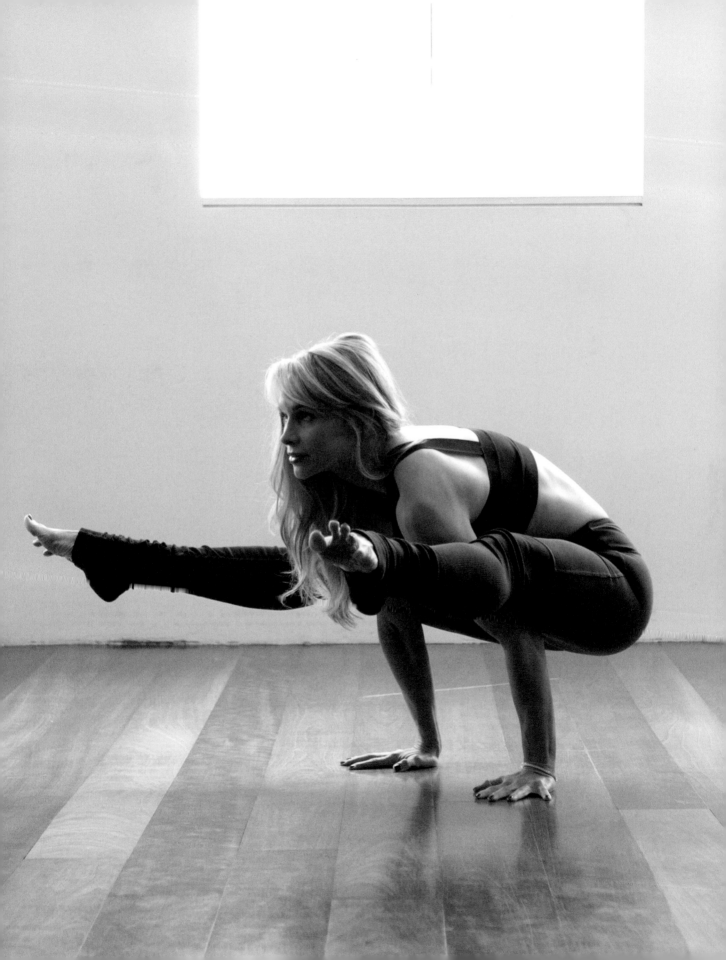

Masumi

LORD OF THE DANCE POSE

• • •

I used to love to do crazy-looking arm balances. One of my favorites doesn't even have a name. I called it Flying Grasshopper. You balance on your palms with one foot on your tricep and the other leg extended behind you.

I can't do it now. I can't put any pressure on my hands. Some days I can't even do Downward Dog.

My yoga has evolved a lot in the past few years, as I have gone through difficult situations.

My daughter, Maia, was born with serious medical problems that ultimately required major surgery when she was eight. She then developed complications that she's still fighting.

After Maia's surgery, while I was staying with her in the hospital, I noticed my left hand felt achy. Then my right knee swelled up like a basketball, and my right hand started hurting. It was really intense pain. I could barely use my hands.

I was used to having pain once in a while in various parts of my body, but it would always pass. My symptoms didn't fit the profile of arthritis or other diseases, so I'd been told I had my own special autoimmune disorder. I had adopted a macrobiotic diet and changed my lifestyle.

It wasn't until I walked into that hospital that the pain began to flare up out of control. I attribute it to stress. I had days where the fear was so intense I could feel myself sweating through my clothing. I had to hide a lot of that; I couldn't let my child see that I was afraid for her.

I now know I have Lyme disease, and that I have probably had it for over ten years.

My relationship with yoga has changed completely. I now understand the philosophy of *aparigraha*, which means nonpossessiveness or nonattachment. I have finally internalized that yoga is about the process, not the outcome. Imagine if I tied my self-worth to my ability to balance on my hands. What would that have done to me?

Today, I try to focus on what I *can* do. I take each day and each circumstance one at a time and try to live my yoga. After all, I spend way more time off my mat than on it.

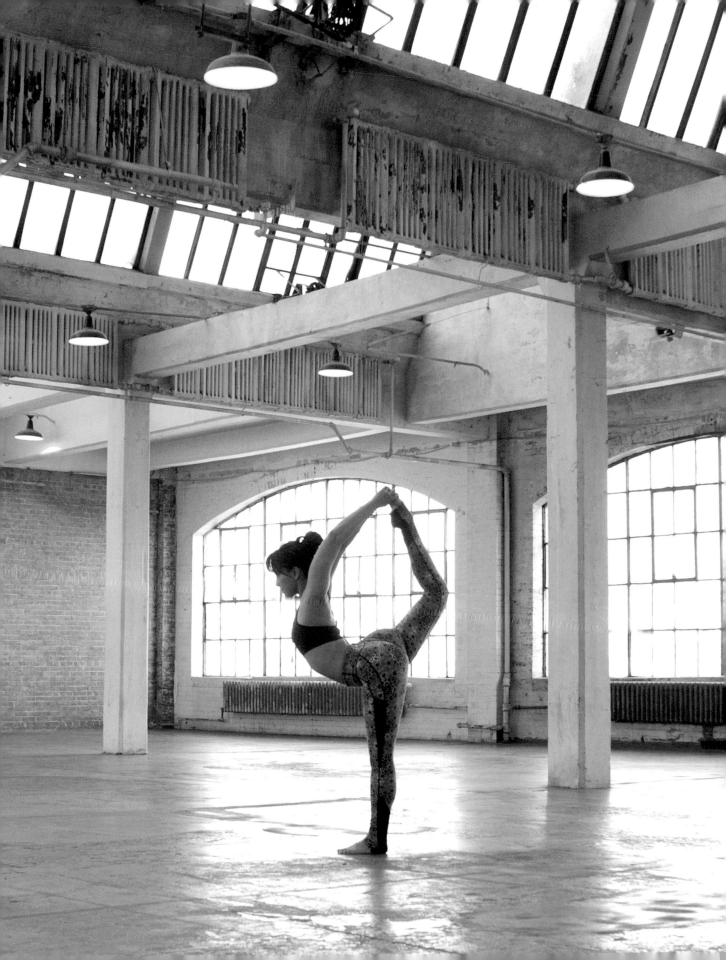

Leo Rising

SCALE POSE

...

When I was twenty-four and told my mom I wanted to change my name to Leo Rising, she said, "Absolutely not." But Leo Rising is who I am. It's my adult name. Now the only people who know my birth name are people who have known me for years.

In astrology, your rising sign is your personality sign. It represents the best qualities that you present to the public, whether you're aware of them or not. My name is my biggest affirmation: *Leo, rise. Leo, go. Leo, show up.*

Astrology, mantras, chakras, the power of manifestation—those things are real for me. I feel like I'm a mystic, that I have always had the ability to sense other levels of consciousness. But I'm also very modern; I love technology and bad reality TV.

Yoga integrates those two sides of me, the extraordinary and the ordinary.

Not everybody wants a workout that's also spiritual, but yoga makes me feel like a whole person.

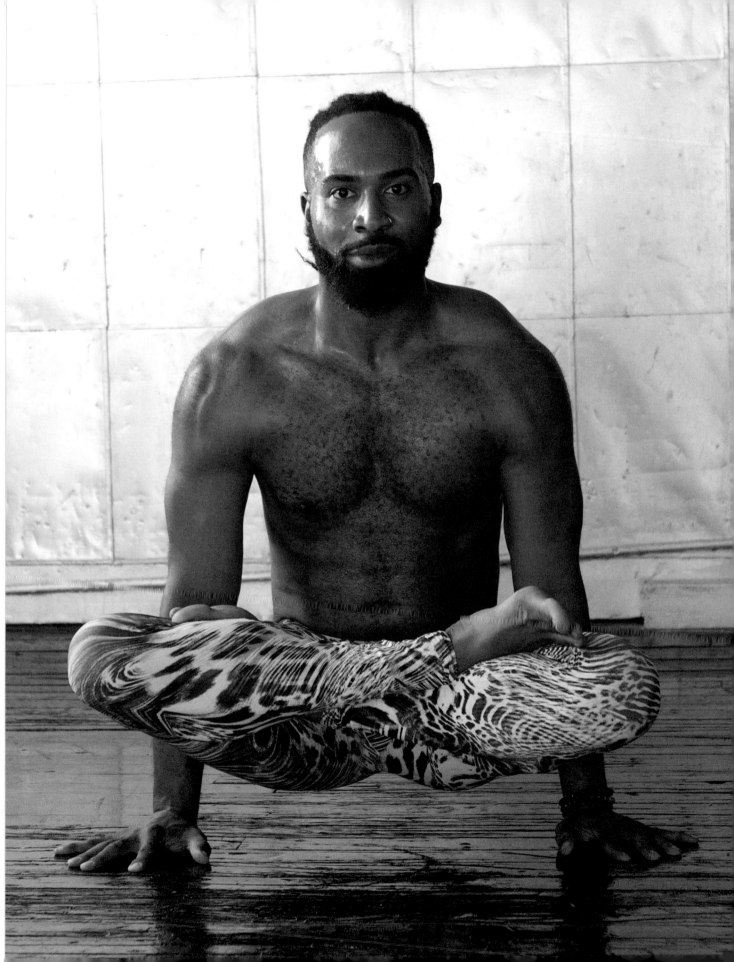

Jim

LEGS-UP-THE-WALL POSE

•••

I live in Boston now, but I grew up surfing in California. There's something very spiritual about surfing. A wave comes; you take off, and you're inside the wave. There's incredible force, but also silence, until the wave crashes and throws you over your board. That's the thrill. That's the rush.

The other thing is, what's underneath the water? You're out there, peaceful, and you see a shadow. What is it? Is it a shark? I thought about that every time I was surfing.

It's the same thing now: fear of the future, fear of the unknown.

So I have cancer, and I'm young. When I found out, the initial news was, my cancer is highly treatable. But there was no discussion of a cure. I figured out pretty quickly that it was very possible I would live a long, normal life and also possible I would die quickly. I took that very hard. I have two little children.

I had found yoga years earlier but done it less often as I got married, had kids, and my job became more busy. But when you get a phone call telling you "You have lymphoma," it's earth-shattering. I had to get back in touch with the spiritual part of my life.

It has taken me a while to get to the other side of fear. Really, I'll never be there. There's no end; it's a daily process.

I ended six months of weekly chemo a week before this photo was taken. It was a targeted, experimental regimen, which is why I still have a full head of hair. As of right now, there is no cancer in my blood. I am in remission. The morning of this photo, I took a yoga class. We were doing inversions—upside-down poses—and when we came out of them, the teacher said, "Land in your feet." I thought, "That's it. Be right here, right now. Be right where you're standing, not where you want to be, not where you were." If I can stay right here and focus on now, the past and the future, for that moment, go away.

Yeah, it's hard. I don't know what's going to happen. But right now I'm living, and I'm so stoked about that.

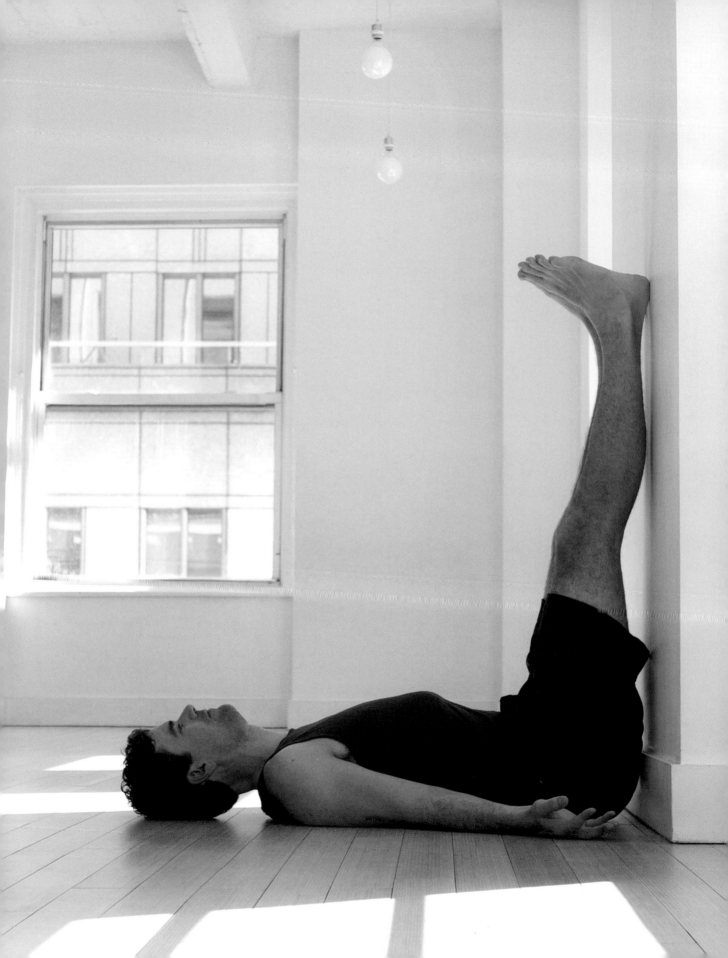

FEATURED IN *YOGA BODIES*

(in order of appearance)

Twee Merrigan, Margarita Manwelyan, Alan Finger, Kimberly Davis Shapiro, Jessamyn Stanley, Betsy Davis, Babette Becker, Kevin Courtney, Marsha Therese Danzig, Jyll Hubbard-Salk, Nayef Zarrour, Bassam Kubba, Mandy Ingber, Loren Fishman, Molly Lehman, Bunny Grossinger, Miles Borrero, Heather Lilleston, Apurva Chokshi, Lauren Mechling, Dana Slamp, Sam Rudra Swartz, Zara Watkins, Crystal McCreary, Victor Colletti, Halle Becker, Karen Maezen Miller, Naomi Watts, Esco Wilson, Loch Baird, Olive Baird, Gus Pallad, Blake Baird, Ava Pesante, Heather Rems Korwin, Michelle Terrell-DeStefano, Shane Farber, Joshua Cohen, Angela Galanti Zambelli, Taryn Toomey, Arvind Saraf, Adesuwa Imasuen, Esosa Imasuen, Claudia Lebenthal, Anna Chung, Chad Dennis, Catie L'Heureux, Jeff Boersma, Dana Flynn, Robyn Burger Schwartz, Sean Nolan, Tommy Nolan, Melissa Pressmar, Tony Richardson, Caroline Williams, Tanya Boulton, Kay Kay Clivio, Luke Beshar, Sheri Celentano, Jim Flemming, Summer Chastant, Jay Graham, Sunny Pallad, Viji Subramaniam, Ryan Kenney, Katherine Rosman, Natalie Ige Muldaur, Benjamin Lorr, Sam Markowitz, Jen Charmatz, Daniela Restivo Delaney, Francesca Valarezo, Clay Twombly, Donna Ng, Susan Everson, Anne Britt, Jeff Bua, Denise Roy, Kiley Holliday, Masumi Goldman, Leo Rising-Scott, Jennilyn Carson, Schuyler Grant, and Jim Wilder.

ACKNOWLEDGMENTS

For believing in *Yoga Bodies*, thank you to Laura Langlie and, from Chronicle Books, Elizabeth Yarborough. For your time, space, generosity, hospitality, expertise, kindness, inspiration, talent and friendship, thank you to Lilly Alexander, Julie Angell, Jennifer Bandier, Anne Britt, Alexandra Brown, Lily Bua, Mary Kay Bua, Yolanda Cazares, Cherry Soda Studios, Dakota Studio, Dune Studios, Downtown Dance Factory, Nicole Eldrige, Michael Gilbert, Sara Golski, Kristi Hein, Rachel Hiles, Ashleigh Hults, Dana James, Anne Kenady, Kett Cosmetics, Steve Kim, Lew Lipton, LightBox-NY, Sheila McKenna, Jamo Mweu, Caroline Novak, Mike Pallad, Ruby Bird Studio, Paul Sunday, Terry Ventre Showroom, Wanderlust Hollywood, and Zara Watkins. Additional thanks to these collaborators whose generous contributions made this book possible: Bandier (women's clothing); PrAna (men's clothing); Nez Jewelry and Chan Luu (jewelry); Cicily Rae (lead makeup and hair), Ivan Betancourt, Jakob Aebly, Jenn Blum, and Charmaine "Charlie" Gibbs-Chiemi (makeup and hair); Jacqueline Moore (wardrobe assistant); Ruby Zolot (production assistant); and Jami Feuerstein (dog trainer). Very special thanks to Jill Arnold Pallad (wardrobe stylist), who contributed well beyond her job description with ingenuity, humor, and boundless enthusiasm.

Thank you to David, as ever, always.
—Lauren Lipton

Thank you to Chip, my sounding board and my beacon. None of this would be possible without you. And to my godmother, Aunty TeTe, I will always "Buy the bathing suit." Loving you!
—Jaimie Baird